What is Disease?

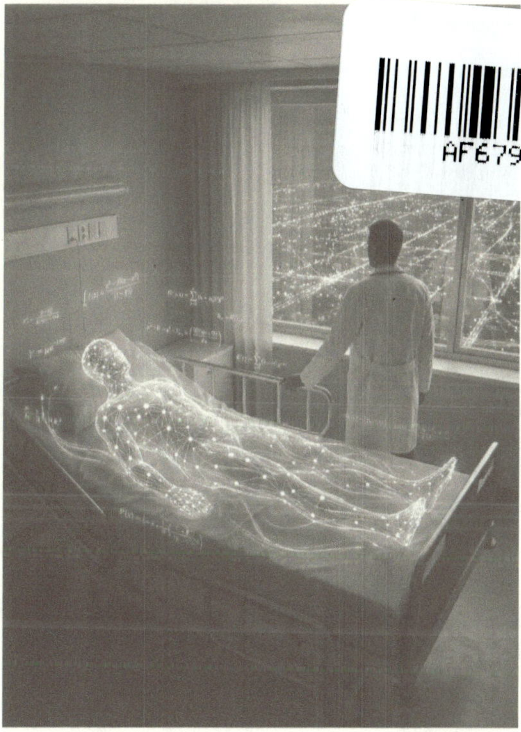

A Unified Theory that explains all Diseases

Dr. Rajkumar Chetty
MBBS MD FRCPath

What is Disease?

Other books by Dr. Rajkumar Chetty

The Myth of the Economy: What Can Nature Teach us That Harvard Does Not
The Puppet Show: How Organisms Dance to the Tune of the Environment
God Molecules: The Biochemistry of God
The Myth of Information Technology: Amazing Wonders of Biological Communication
The Myth of Human Intelligence: Nature's Incredible Ways of Problem-Solving
The Universe as a Complex System: What Can Modern Science and Eastern Philosophy Tell Us About Order, Creation, God and Religion?
The Secret Lives of Microbes: The Good, the Bad and the Ugly

Print ISBN 978-1-960405-69-2
ebook ISBN 978-1-960405-70-8

Cover Design by Guy D. Corp
www.GrafixCorp.com

STAIRWAY PRESS

www.StairwayPress.com
1000 West Apache Trail
Suite 126
Apache Junction, AZ 85120 USA

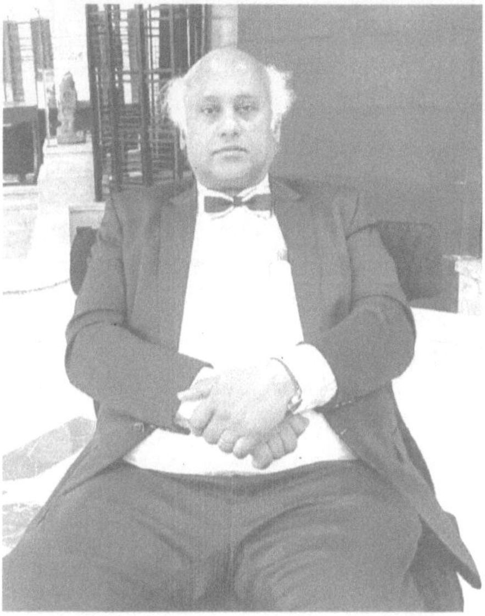

About Dr. Chetty

DR. RAJKUMAR CHETTY is an Indian British medical doctor. After completing his medical education, he specialized in Clinical Biochemistry and Pharmaceutical Medicine and currently works as the Head of Medical Laboratory Services at a hospital in Dubai.

He is a Fellow of the Royal College of Pathologists, United Kingdom. Dr. Chetty is also a Fellow of the Faculty of Pharmaceutical Medicine, Royal College of Physicians, UK. He has worked for the National Health Service UK for many years as a Chemical Pathologist. He spent over seven years working in Pharmaceutical R&D at the global pharmaceutical company AstraZeneca at their Alderley Park research facility near Manchester. During this time, he was involved in many clinical trials of new drugs as a Principal Investigator.

Dr. Chetty is registered with the General Medical Council UK as a specialist in two medical specialties—Clinical Biochemistry and Pharmaceutical Medicine. In total he has more than 35 years of professional experience in hospital practice, teaching, and research gained in India, United Kingdom, Saudi Arabia, and UAE.

Dr. Chetty has a deep-rooted interest in scientific philosophy and revels in thinking, writing and talking about profound worldly phenomena and their scientific basis. In terms of writing experience Dr. Chetty has published five books in his native language of Tamil on the topic of scientific basis of spirituality. He has also published seven eBooks in English on a variety of topics touching upon spiritualism, economics, information science, medicine and philosophy. His most recent book in print version, published by Stairway Press, is *The Secret World of the Microbes: the Good, the Bad and the Ugly*.

More of his works are awaiting publication.

Contents

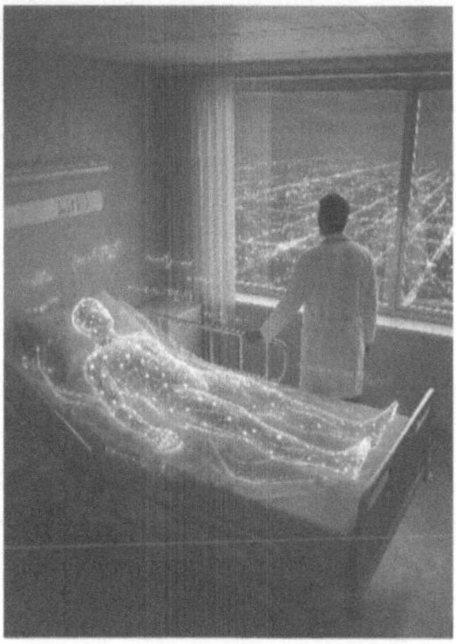

1. Introduction: What is Disease

THE AUTHOR DR Rajkumar Chetty is a medical doctor who has specialised in Chemical Pathology and Pharmaceutical Medicine and has over 35 years of experience in the field of medicine gained across India, United Kingdom, Saudi Arabia and the United Arab Emirates. With his breadth of knowledge and experience he has attempted to unravel the phenomenon of diseases with a view to conceptualize our understanding rather than simply follow the traditional descriptive path. His approach is a significant departure from the conventional thinking on the nature of human diseases.

Combating diseases is an innate biological characteristic. This is because even animals have this natural tendency to seek medicinal substances to cure their diseases. That is why we need to really understand the phenomenon of diseases from a more fundamental level. What is its place in the universe? Why are all multi-cellular life forms suffering from diseases? What is disease? Is it a disorder, as opposed to order, speaking in thermodynamic terms? Are we prone to disorder, in other words disease, just as any other thermodynamic system? Are we spending free energy and resources to maintain a state of order in the body while the body as a thermodynamic system constantly tries to move towards a state of disorder? Is disease a warning that individual human life system is beginning to fail to maintain order, allowing the thermodynamic laws to take over, and moves us towards a point of no return viz. death? It sounds like fighting disease is an evolutionary characteristic of life systems not limited to human beings.

For that matter, life systems spend an enormous amount of energy to keep disorder away. To maintain the state of life we, as well as other life systems, must create order at considerable expense to the point where a logical question arises – why life? If the life principles, i.e., the sum of all biochemical processes inside a life system do not work against disorder then the body will move inexorably towards a state of disorder as mandated by the second law of thermodynamics. Disease can possibly represent states of inadequacy where the body struggles to keep disorder away. This may be because the life processes that keep the dance of life alive, start failing in a localized or global manner. Death ensues when the failures reach a point where the disorder takes the upper hand. The rapid rate of degradation of a dead body represents the natural force that was constantly trying to destroy life. It is the law of the Universe.

There should be a way of bringing all human diseases under one unifying principle just like Einstein sought a 'Unified Field Theory' till his death. The author views diseases more as a physicochemical phenomenon rather than a simple biological one. There is a lot of chemistry and physics beneath the biology of human diseases. That makes it even more interesting.

The author likens diseases to sociological ills and proposes that human diseases are 'social' problems of the 'cellular society'. There is not much difference between diseases and social maladies which he has explained in a convincing way. Human 'cellular society' suffers from the same ills as the real society of humans. That means the answers to social issues could be found in the way doctors treat diseases. Or you could turn it around and say doctors must treat the diseases the way sociologists and policy makers address social ills.

The author states that huge multicellular organisms are vulnerable to cellular disorder and humans are no exception. The human body is estimated to contain tens of trillions of cells, which perform tasks according to their structural and functional specialisation. They function as one whole because they are inter-linked by a communication network, the complexity of which is mind-boggling and still not completely understood. Information transfer is central to the process of metabolic control and cells constantly exchange information with regards to fuel levels, blood pressure, nutrient concentrations, oxygen, minerals like sodium, potassium, calcium, phosphate, magnesium etc. and any deviation in the internal environment is attended by compensatory mechanisms that will restore the constancy. Invariably, these adaptive mechanisms require a chain of communication between effectors and target cells, often involving several cell types.

Physical, biological or chemical insults can lead to difficulties in cellular communication which can be localised to a particular organ or to a limited number of cell types, or can be widespread affecting multiple or, where death is imminent, all cell types. The resultant phenomenon is disease. Death is the final state in the evolution of the disease where the coherent functioning of all cells is no longer feasible due to global information failure. When the adaptive mechanisms of homeostasis fail, due to failure of one or more cell types to either generate or respond to informational molecules, the outcome is a disorderly state that is not responsive to the internal nor the external environment of the body. The author calls this state as disease and the body as a system will manifest biochemical and clinical features that are diagnostic.

The author explores the concept of disease from a biological perspective viewing it as a failure to maintain the constancy of the internal environment of the body due to defects in intercellular communication. He has shown that diverse disease-causing mechanisms produce convergent effects on key biochemical processes to bring about global disruption in the communication capabilities of the cells. He has also attempted to show that multi-cellular life systems like humans, consisting of trillions of cells, are vulnerable to cellular disorder because of this breakdown of information transfer resulting in an inability to function as a cohesive unit. In summary, he claims that information failure is the basis of cellular disorder associated with all human diseases.

The author draws heavily on Claude Shannon's seminal paper published in 1948 that defined information and helped formulate a mathematical theory on communication. Basically, a typical communication system, as described by Shannon, consists of a message source, a coder to encrypt the information, a channel for communication, and finally a decoder to receive the information. His information theory was developed to understand the transmission of electronic signals. But this theory now has had an impact on biology as well, particularly with reference to DNA, because of the obvious relationship between DNA and biological information.

Based on the concept of Shannon's model, it can be deduced that errors in information transmission within the human body can occur due to Defects in information source, Coding, transmission and channel errors and Decoding (Receiver) errors.

The author has meticulously categorized all known diseases under these three headings. This is an incredibly different way of classifying diseases. No textbooks on medicine have taken this approach to understanding or describing diseases. This is the most unique selling point of this book. The author challenges anyone who can point out a disease that cannot be fitted into this framework. In one full chapter the author examines the nature of drugs currently in use and the focus of pharmaceutical research for future drugs. The detailed description of all types of medicines used in modern times clearly points to one single striking fact: they all act by interfering with cellular information transfer of some sort. There is no exception. This vindicates the author's argument that human diseases are the result of failure or altered information exchange between cells.

Based on the assumption that diseases are failures in information transfer between cells, the author claims that the phenomenon of disease should be unique to only multi-cellular life forms, and not unicellular life. For that matter, even (natural) death should be a unique multi-cellular life property. Unicellular microbes endlessly divide into daughter cells in the presence of adequate nutrient supply and so do cancer cells, which behave autonomously much like unicellular life.

Moving on, the author argues that it is not a secret that more than half of medicines used by us in the practice of modern medicine are plant products, or those made by lowly fungi. It is an interesting point to discuss why nature has evolved medicinal substances. One could surmise that they exist to restore order and balance in life systems. Many of these medicinal substances may be made by plants, shrubs and microbes for their own needs including defence but one cannot discount the theory that they are there to help maintain orderly function in multicellular life systems. Plants are the groceries or supermarkets that Nature has created in a non-profitable sense where life systems can 'shop' for their food and medicines. It is intriguing that nature has evolved medicinal substances that are made by other life systems that help in curing diseases. This puts the concept of disease in a philosophical dimension.

Lung diseases are like crisis in gas supply. Lungs are unable to import oxygen from the environment. Same problem can hit us from related causes like low levels of Haemoglobin and red cells in the blood. Red cells are our 'Oxygen tankers'. Problems with red cells will devastate us no different from what would happen to your industrial economy if your oil tankers got hit. You might think nothing will happen if trucks and tankers go off the road. You are very wrong. You will be surprised how quickly your petrol stations will dry out. You will be stunned to see empty supermarket shelves too soon for your comfort.

We have come to believe that we live in a society where science and technology have made our lives invincible. This is not true. Our society is as fragile as our body. It takes only three minutes of anoxia (lack of oxygen) for you to kick your bucket irrespective of the fact how rich you are or how much food energy you have in your body. We are that fragile. That is why when there is a heart attack or respiratory failure the cellular tankers carrying food and oxygen are stuck in the blood vessels like your vehicles getting stuck on the roads due to roadblocks. It is a roller-coaster ride soon after that and before you know it you are gone. You are on your way to find housing in a cemetery. Your maker awaits!

Cancer is a killer. We are all afraid of it. Why is it so deadly? What kind of disease is it? Cancer is likened by the author to capitalistic societies. This is all about unequal sharing of resources. Greedy cells take over the entire supply of resources without regard to the needs of normal cells. This is a typical characteristic of cancer cells. If you look carefully that is what capitalistic bosses do. They have little time to think about the millions of people who have nothing or, at best, have very little. Doctors treat cancers by surgically excising the cancerous tissue and throwing it out. Or use chemotherapy or radiation to kill the greedy cancer cells. All this vigour in treating greediness is evidently absent when it comes to economy in our society. This is a lesson for us to learn to solve the sociological problem of wealth inequality.

Doctors, especially those practising acute medicine, know only too well that patients admitted for various illnesses often progress through strikingly similar course in the end. This phenomenon has been described as the 'final common pathway of disease and death'. What the above phenomena indicates is that there is convergence in disease pathways despite the diversity in aetiology. This interesting fact has not been explored adequately in medical literature. There is a whole chapter aiming to unravel the underlying mechanisms of this convergence.

In simple words one could say that when a person suffers from a disease the destination is always death. People may begin the journey from different starting points. But at some point, the journey starts converging into a single highway that takes you to the 'City of Death'. There is a saying 'all roads lead to Rome'. In medical parlance we can revise this saying as 'all diseases lead to death'. May be some roads could be small, narrow roads and so could take a longer time to reach the destination. The author supposes this is like the chronic, non-acute type of diseases that is not a fast superhighway to death. In some cases, the disease is acute and can take you swiftly to your destination in no time.

The point the author tries to drive home is that whatever roads you begin your journey on will not matter after some point. All these roads will begin to converge on a small set of roads which will eventually end up in one final route. This is the final common pathway.

The primary aetiological agent and the pathogenic mechanism(s) of the primary disease of a dying patient could have been one of hundreds of known causes of disease in man but, after the initial insult to the system through biological, physical or chemical agents, which resulted in a disease, the subsequent course of events in most if not all diseases are surprisingly not specific to the disease at all. This is true in both acute and non-acute illnesses. This is truly a remarkable finding in medical practice that might have surprised most doctors, especially those who practice acute medicine.

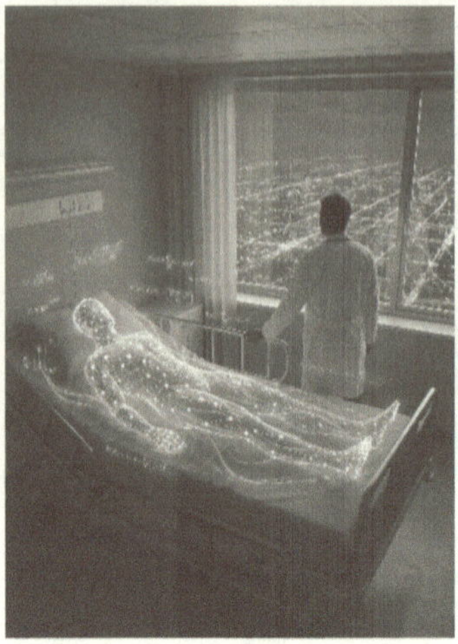

2. Living and Non-Living Systems are Error-Prone by Nature

IN THIS BOOK, Dr. Rajkumar Chetty advances a simple but radical thesis: all human diseases can be understood as failures of information flow and error-control within the "cellular society" that makes up the body. By treating diseases not only as biochemical events but as breakdowns in communication, coordination, and order across trillions of interacting cells, he offers a unified way to think about conditions that are usually taught in isolation—infectious, genetic, autoimmune, degenerative, and even so-called "lifestyle" diseases.

This perspective invites clinicians, scientists, and thoughtful lay readers to step back from protocols and organ systems and instead ask how life maintains order against constant error, and what happens—biologically, socially, and economically—when those error-correction systems begin to fail.

Humanity spent 8.8 trillion dollars on health in the year 2021. This is the total spending on health by all nations combined. Cost of medicines alone accounts for 0.5 trillion dollars annually and the rest covers all other aspects of healthcare provision. This could include building hospitals, salaries for healthcare workers, diagnostic tests, medical and surgical procedures, etc. This amounts to almost 10% of global GDP, which was estimated to be around 85 trillion dollars in the year 2020. We can safely say we spend one-tenth of our global income on health.

Free healthcare is considered a birthright in many countries. People living in other countries are not so fortunate and have to fork out high levels of insurance premiums to cover their healthcare. Why those countries do not use tax revenue to provide free healthcare is a political question outside the scope of this book.

Health obviously ranks very high on the global agenda irrespective of national differences. Nations focus on delivery of good healthcare, private or public, to their citizens because a healthy population is vital for a productive society.

Why should we be healthy? It sounds like a stupid question to ask because, obviously, health is better than unhealth. There is still a quite significant proportion of the world's population who do not have access to good healthcare due to either the high costs or lack of infrastructure like hospitals.

Why do we fight disease at such a high cost?

Diseases cause pain and suffering and rob individuals and societies of their productivity. The urge to stay healthy is an innate human characteristic. Today, in many parts of the world, going to the doctor at the slightest sign of discomfort is routine and seeking medical attention when we are ill is now taken for granted. Yet until the 1800s most humans lived without the luxury of hospitals and modern doctors. That does not mean our ancestors were passive in the face of illness. Across cultures, numerous ancient medical practices have been documented, showing that humans have always tried to cure disease using the accumulated wisdom of previous generations. Remarkably, many of these practices have since been shown to have real scientific value, and some are still used—and studied—today.

Our body has powerful defensive, self-healing, regenerative properties. In many cases, what doctors do to cure disease is actually supported—and sometimes made possible—by these built-in repair mechanisms. In that sense, doctors may occasionally claim credit that truly belongs to the body's own regenerative capacity.

Billions of dollars spent to combat COVID-19 produced less overall benefit compared to the natural immunity our bodies developed toward the virus. Our immune system fought COVID-19, and no one can count the cost of it, let alone quantify the number of lives saved. If the internal immune defense was unavailable, a substantial proportion of the world's population might have been at risk. The early fatality rate of 2-3% was low because our immune system helped us fight it. If our immune system was not there, we would have succumbed to the virus in masses. What we achieved with trillions of dollars at the societal level (diagnostic tests, vaccines, hospitalized care) was achieved by our own bodies internally at no cost. Fighting diseases is not an activity stemming from our modernization, or intelligence, or availability of money and resources, but an intrinsic phenomenon which throws a different light on the subject.

Apart from COVID infections there are hundreds of other infectious diseases that afflict humans. Our immune systems play a big role in fighting them and we hardly ever thank it. We believe it was the antibiotics and other treatments given by the doctor that helped us fight the infections. That is a totally incorrect understanding stemming from the lack of fundamental understanding of diseases. Few thought our immune system waged a war on the invading microbe at a considerable biological cost. This takes a toll on the internal body economy of the individual life system. The benefit of this biological war is the recovery from our infections. Without our internal immune system, outcomes of external medical treatment would be far less impressive. Our immune system subsidizes the cost of medical treatment significantly.

If you think it is only our immune system that offers "free healthcare," you are wrong. Antibiotics doctors prescribe are the intellectual property rights of fungi and other lifeforms. Why should fungi make the antibiotics that you and I use to treat infectious diseases?

Combating diseases is an innate biological characteristic because even animals have this natural tendency to seek medicinal substances to cure their diseases. The author shows in a later chapter how many different types of animals seek out medicinal substances to cure their ailments. This may seem unbelievable. How can animals know what plants or herbs to consume when they are ill? We think we need pharmacists and organic chemists to tell us. It sounds like fighting disease is an evolutionary characteristic of life systems not limited to human beings.

That is why we need to really understand the phenomenon of diseases from a more fundamental level. What is its place in the universe? Why do all multicellular life forms suffer from diseases? What is disease? Speaking in thermodynamic terms, is it a disorder, as opposed to order? Are we prone to disorder—in other words disease—just as any other thermodynamic system? Do we spend energy and resources to maintain a state of order in the body while the body as a thermodynamic system constantly tries to move toward a state of disorder? Is disease a warning that the individual human life system is failing to maintain order, allowing the thermodynamic laws to take over, and moving us toward a point of no return, viz. death?

For that matter, life systems spend an enormous amount of energy to keep disorder away. To maintain the state of life, we, as well as other life systems, must create order at considerable expense to the point where a logical question arises: why life?

If the life principles— i.e. the sum of all biochemical processes inside a life system—do not work against disorder, then the body will move inexorably toward a state of disorder as mandated by the second law of thermodynamics. Disease can possibly represent states of inadequacy where the body struggles to keep disorder away. This may be because the life processes that keep the dance of life alive start failing in a localized or global manner. Death ensues when the failures reach a point where the disorder takes the upper hand. The rapid rate of degradation of a dead body represents the natural force that was constantly trying to destroy life.

It is a law of the universe.

A disease is like having a device or equipment at home that does not work well. A faulty appliance can be considered useless as we don't get the benefit of its function anymore. Sometimes a faulty appliance or equipment can cause accidents, particularly the electrical and heavy-duty kind of equipment. So, we spend a fortune on repairing the faulty equipment. If we count the cost of the annual expenditure across the globe on repair and maintenance of machines it is likely to be quite high, and I do not think anyone has worked out these kinds of statistics yet. It is the "healthcare" spend for our machines!

We spend a lot on maintenance of our cars. Consumers demand a warranty for the appliances they buy. It could be one, two, or more years. This applies to cars, electronic equipment, and all sorts of devices. We cannot unfortunately ask for "warranty" for a healthy human being from our creator!

You get what you get.

We have the luxury of demanding warranty for our machines, and the manufacturers accede to this demand invariably because the consumer will refuse to buy a device that will break down all the time, potentially leading to high costs of repair to the consumer. The warranty issued by the manufacturer does not mean that the appliance will work without any fault forever. It means that the manufacturer will meet the cost of the repairs and the consumer does not have to pay. This is like the free healthcare given to the citizens, but the provision of free healthcare does not mean the government will pay for it. You pay for it indirectly through your taxes.

Machines and the human body both will develop faults at some point and this can happen at any stage of life. A new device that fails straight out of the box is like a birth defect in a baby—both resemble production-line faults. With machines we can issue a product recall or arrange for a replacement; with congenital birth defects we do not have that option. In such cases, only God can "recall" a human life.

Aging machines are prone to faults much like our elderly population. Wear and tear are not unique to machines. Human bodies succumb to the same fate. Many of the human diseases set in at predictable ages. Arthritis is a disease that creeps in during mid-life only. It is rarely seen in young children. The constant burden of weight-bearing and use over decades leads to joint inflammation and degradation in an aging human. At some point the machines get worn out to the extent they stop working. Our human body reaches a similar fate roughly after about 60-80 years, give or take. Death depicts the permanent retirement of the human body. Our body is condemned like old appliances arriving at a landfill.

Human machines are more error-prone than industrial machines going by the incidence of so many types of diseases that affect us humans. Maybe the cosmic engineering that created life was not good enough. Or it could be that the user maintenance of the "human machine" is no good. We ill-treat our body "machines" by not taking good care of them. A machine's manufacturer expects the user to follow proper instructions when using and operating the machines.

A car that was serviced regularly has less chance of a breakdown. Many manufacturers and insurers put a clause in the contracts that the user agrees to maintain the machines as per recommended guidelines, failing which the user loses the right to claim compensation.

Unfortunately, users of the "human machines" often neglect the service and maintenance part. We overeat and become obese.

We do not put our muscles to work, relying on tools and engines to do the tasks. We expose ourselves to all kinds of environmental toxins thanks to our industrialization. We eat highly processed unnatural foods, omitting the natural vegetables and fruits. We expose our body machines to insults like alcohol and drugs.

How can we then expect a healthy life?

A more likely explanation for the high incidence of diseases we suffer could be not the fault of God's engineering design but user maintenance issues. Maybe we are pampered by healthcare service providers too much. Strangely, could we sue hospitals and doctors if we feel we have not been diagnosed and treated correctly?

Our knowledge about diseases has grown over the centuries and probably millennia. We could catalogue all known human diseases and trace the chronology of when we first understood each of those diseases. We did not know about microbes until the 1800s when the use of microscopes helped to identify tiny enemies.

We did not know about genetic diseases until the late 20th century because the structure of DNA was discovered in 1953, shortly after which the gene sequencing technique discovered by Frederick Sanger emerged. Only in the late 20th century did the human genome sequencing project unveil a whole lot of information about human gene codes and what goes wrong in many diseases. Many diseases previously thought to be unrelated to genes are now known to have a genetic basis. Diseases are now seen as faults in programming codes much like our digital machines. This throws an entirely new light on the nature of human diseases.

Our increasingly inactive lifestyle has led to the origin of many lifestyle diseases which we are now grappling with. Exposure to man-made chemicals and pollutants has led to the rise in many cancers and other diseases. Our body is as prone to environmental pollution as our lands. Many types of lung diseases are due to airborne pollutants, which means that new diseases have been appearing after the onset of our industrialization. That means that diseases are not static entities that have always existed all the time.

Diseases can be created too.

Doctors read about these diseases in medical schools, but their teaching is not geared to provide a fundamental understanding of human disease. Instead, the teaching is restricted to reductionist approaches and there is never any chance of a unified understanding of the diseases.

Why do we need a unified understanding of the disease phenomenon? If medical sciences work adequately well, then why bother? People get cured and lives are saved. What is the issue?

There is no effort to find the common motifs underlying human diseases. The author wants to philosophize on the nature of human diseases. My desire is like the need for art. There is no real reason, or need, for art, but art makes life more beautiful. It is the joy of thinking. There are thousands of medical textbooks and an equal number of medical journals. They serve a purpose severely limited by conservatism and orthodoxy. This book takes a different approach and takes an offbeat road toward the discovery of the fundamental causative principles underlying the phenomenon of human disease.

It may not shatter the world but hopefully will offer some very interesting reading for interested readers, medics and nonmedics alike. My hope is that it will attract the interest of information scientists, engineers, cybernetic theorists, and sociologists too.

There should be a way of bringing all human diseases under one unifying principle like Einstein seeking a "Unified Field Theory" till his death. I view diseases more as a physicochemical phenomenon rather than a simple, biological one. There is a lot of chemistry and physics beneath the biology of human diseases. That makes it even more interesting.

The human body is a society of cells. The trillions of cells inside the human body must cooperate, communicate, and contribute to the cause of the survival of the human body as a whole. Regulating the function of 30 trillion cells is no joke. We are just 8 billion people on the planet divided into 196 countries in comparison. As a human society can we consider ourselves successful in maintaining fairness, order, peace, and cooperation?

The answer is a resounding no.

We have lost count of the number of wars fought killing our own kind. Wars remind me of the many autoimmune diseases humans suffer from. Some common examples include rheumatoid arthritis, lupus, etc. The feature of the autoimmune diseases is self-mediated attack on your own self. Metaphorically speaking, the human society surely is afflicted with quite rampant autoimmune "diseases,"

We have an unjust way of sharing natural resources. Inequality in wealth ticks like a time bomb waiting to explode. To me, war, terrorism, and destruction are much like the autoimmune diseases that our bodies encounter.

Inequality in sharing resources and wealth leads to poverty and hunger, which to me looks so much like malnutrition of the body. Greedy accumulation of wealth by a few, at the expense of most of the population, is reminiscent of the way cancerous diseases work. Looking at the situation, I conclude that our human society is very ill and afflicted with many "diseases" which we may call by a different term: social problems. Will our society survive the social diseases? Or has it reached the stage of irreversible deterioration that can only be met with the "death" of the society?

I liken diseases to sociological ills because I propose that human diseases are "social" problems of the "cellular society." I do not think there is much difference between diseases and social maladies, which I have explained later hopefully in a convincing way. National problems increase in proportion to the population increase. The problem in our society is largely due to the excessive population and the demands placed on resource allocation, crime monitoring, competition for jobs, hunger, poverty, education, etc., which have created sociological issues that are akin to diseases. Human "cellular society" suffers from the same ills as the real society of humans. That means the answers to social issues could be found in the way doctors treat diseases. Or you could turn it around and say doctors must treat diseases the way sociologists and policymakers address social ills.

One of the challenges of multiple interacting units within a complex system is internal communication. This is even more important when you have 30 trillion of them! How do they stay in contact with each other? How do they know what they need to do and when? Amazingly, an intricate network of communication channels and mechanisms operate inside our body to achieve this near-impossible feat.

But, as always, communication can fail. Even inside a small office there can be chaos when systems are down, and you can imagine what will happen when there is downtime (temporary or permanent) in cellular communication channels inside the body.

For example, polio is a disease of the nerves where a virus damaged information conduction channels. This is an obvious example; there are hundreds of such disorders in communication channels inside the body. Invariably, each communication disruption leads to diseases. This makes me wonder if communication failure between cells is a unifying feature of all faults in the human "machines"—a fault we call disease.

If we take seriously the idea that disease is the social pathology of our cellular society, then our approach to medicine and health policy can no longer be limited to suppressing isolated symptoms or targeting single molecules.

Clinicians may begin to see familiar disorders as manifestations of deeper communication failures in the organism; researchers may look for unifying information-theoretic principles beneath diverse pathologies; and lay readers may recognize how their daily choices either support or sabotage the body's fragile order-maintaining machinery.

My hope is that the framework developed in the chapters that follow will not only change how we classify diseases, but also how we design therapies, allocate resources, and imagine a healthier relationship between individual bodies and the societies we inhabit.

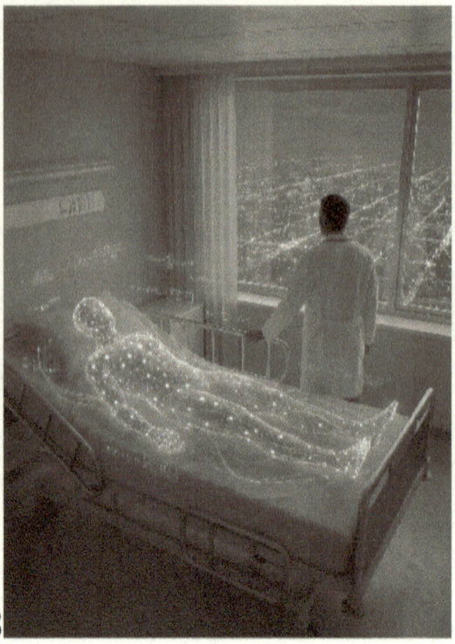

8

3. A Systems View of Diseases

IN 1944, ERWIN Schrodinger wrote a masterpiece called *What is Life?* This was a rather small book but looked at the phenomenon of life from a physicist's point of view. That was an amazing piece of work because no one had done that before and was certainly not expected from a physicist. Remember that it was the time we did not even know how life forms used information for day-to-day metabolism and for heredity. For that reason, this piece of writing won critical acclaim at that time.

Today inter-disciplinary research is commonplace and biologists, chemists, mathematicians and physicists work together. This book is an attempt in that direction. I want to explore the phenomenon of disease from a different vantage point; I want to forget I am a doctor and de-learn what I have been taught from standard medical texts. I want to offer a different concept of diseases—ignoring conventional boundaries of medical specialties.

Describing all signs and symptoms of diseases, their causes, and their treatments is enough for the practice of medicine. But isn't there any scope for looking at diseases from a dynamic, systemic viewpoint? If a physicist looked at the human body as a complex adaptive system, how would they understand the phenomenon of disease? If an engineer looked at the human body as an intricately designed, multi-component system with numerous control devices, would he or she be able to understand disease from a cybernetic point of view? If a biologist looked at the human body as an ecosystem consisting of multiple types of cellular species, would different answers for the concept of disease be found? If an Information technologist viewed the human body as a society of cells, dependent on information, then what would be the take on disorder amongst the cells? What would disease be called?

A disease can be considered as a disorderly state inside your body; there is a problem affecting the orderly function of the human body—which might last for a short period or until you cease to exist. No human is an exception. Without doubt, all of us at some point or other in our lives will develop illnesses. This suggests our body as a system is prone to disorder. To be honest, it is very true. I am sure there is no machine in the world that works without fault all its life. Bio systems are no exception. They are susceptible to malfunction.

Diseases are malfunctions of your body.

In principle they are no different from malfunctions in your gadgets. Repair of your gadgets by mechanics and engineers requires time. The error must be identified and a solution found for fixing it. Professional mechanics have tools for 'diagnosing' the 'disease' of the machine and have established guidelines for fixing the faults.

Doctors are mechanics for the body.

They spend years studying and training to become doctors. They must study in detail about body physiology and pathology of diseases. The only difference between doctors and gadget mechanics is life and death. A mistake by a doctor can mean the end for the patient. This is an irreplaceable mistake. But mechanics dealing with machines can afford to take their own time and need not worry too much about fatal outcomes. Nobody will weep over a dead machine, will they? We also must remember that we do not worry too much about very old machines 'dying' because we all know that machines have a life span. We do not expect machines to work longer than 8-10 years on average. But, on the contrary, humans are unable to accept the inevitability of death that occurs due to old age and the consequent wear and tear of the body. Nowadays, we consider death at ages in the region of 70 years as untimely and cannot come to terms with it.

One of the other unusual aspects of medical profession is that they face the wrath of the public when a patient cannot be saved. The relatives of the dead patient, or harmed patient, can hold the doctor in court for damages. We hardly do that to our mechanics, do we? No wonder doctors pay huge premiums for malpractice insurances to defend them.

My idea of discussing this similarity between a mechanic and a doctor is only to show that diseases are fundamentally systemic faults. Advances in medical sciences over the last 50 years have enriched our knowledge about human diseases. Human Genome sequencing projects are poised to throw open the gates for more knowledge about our diseases. This is all exciting, no doubt. But, truly, do we know about the true nature of disease? Of course, we do but I have my own doubts about whether we really have grasped the deeper meanings of the concept of disease.

I am a medical doctor and have also specialised in Biochemistry and Pharmaceutical medicine. My belief is that medical sciences promoted a reductionist thinking for too long. There is no doubt it is necessary to understand the precise, molecular and cellular basis of the disease phenomenon, but unfortunately, modern medicine drowned itself in too much detail. Conceptualization went missing. There is no attempt to philosophize about the nature of diseases.

This is sad.

Systemic disorder is not unique to human body. Any system

comprised of multiple and dissimilar components is prone to disorder.

Our society is like the human body in that there are billions of human beings working together—just as billions of cells work together inside the human body. Sociologists and economists try to solve the maladies that affect the society: poverty, unemployment, civil unrest, terrorism, overpopulation, illiteracy and debt, etc. In my view, all of these social maladies are conceptually similar to the diseases that affect our body. Each type of malady has a variety of causes and solutions. Identifying social disorders is one thing, but it is a different ball game when it comes to finding a remedy that works.

Moreover, it is not difficult to see that many of social problems like poverty, illiteracy, unemployment, etc. have a relation to each other and may even have a common cause that needs to be addressed rather than each one at a time. Eradication of the root cause may alleviate many social ills. This is systemic thinking. That is the difference between macroeconomics and microeconomics. It is this principle I want to apply to the understanding of human diseases. I want to look at the forest and not the trees.

What I mean is that a headache or body pain or fever can be treated simply with a pain killer. This certainly relieves the immediate problem. But it does not help prevent recurrence of the same problem or growth of the problem if the patient had an underlying illness. If the doctor does not bother about these considerations, then he has failed in his duty—just as politicians and sociologists fail when they address social problems superficially. Unrest or protest warns sociologists of some problem. Dealing with protesters with police action and arrest may help solve the problem temporarily, but will it help in the long-term?

What I feel, as a practising doctor, is that we need serious insights into the broad principles of human disease. There is a craving amongst many medical professionals for more of concepts and less of details. I have hardly seen any articles in medical literature in the last few decades that looks at a holistic view of human diseases cutting across organ systems. In fact, I do not recall any. What is the reason? What is happening? Is there something wrong here?

Let us go back to the example of social ills. I am sure there are many articles and books being written about the social problems I listed above. There are, in addition, television debates as well. Economists, politicians, sociologists and people from other disciplines write and talk about these problems and there is a general sense of a broad-based thinking here. This is missing in medicine. This is my worry. Why can't there be a broad synthesis of medical knowledge out of seemingly disparate and needlessly detailed minutiae?

Modern medical students are bewildered by the number of diseases and syndromes and there is a widely held belief that medical science is very complicated and unwieldy and hence springs the need for increasing sub-specialisation. Nowadays it is the norm to see a specialist for your illnesses—and there are specialists for heart, kidneys, lungs, brains and so on. Each organ speciality has much information pouring in as a result of medical research. This leads to further sub-specialisation. No doctor can hope to know all about the minute details about all human diseases.

In fact, doctors these days are reluctant to venture beyond the boundaries of their own medical specialty and do not hesitate to refer their patients to other specialists at the earliest suspicion of involvement of another organ system! Specialist doctors have a narrow view of their patients and are often unable to look at the whole simply because of the way medical sciences evolved and the way medical practice itself evolved. Sometimes it can be days or weeks before you see another specialist, having seen one before, and if someone has many complaints then he or she might see many different specialists at varying points in time.

It is common for some information to be missed by the doctors if there are multiple medical conditions for the same patient. Moreover, many medicines have side effects and some are incompatible with other medicines. The doctors cannot know all about these drug-drug interactions and incompatibilities. This might mean patients could be put on medicines that should not be used together. Wrong prescriptions account for a substantial amount of iatrogenic harm.

Modern medicine is a descriptive science. Diseases are described to minute detail and doctors are trained to look at diseases like a detective trying to solve a mystery. The doctor collects more evidence by way of diagnostic tests and symptoms and signs. The aim of the doctor is to narrow down the 'suspects' and do more tests to confirm the diagnosis.

In most cases this works.

But there are still several diseases where the diagnosis is hard. It is like unsolved crimes. In many patients, the diagnosis is never made even until death. In some countries, undiagnosed death should be followed by a post-mortem examination to help uncover the missed diagnosis. This obviously helps the relatives to know the cause of the death, but also has enormous educational value to the doctor and his team. This is different from the need for forensic evidence which also requires post-mortem examinations. Whether it is for forensic detective work or for nailing the diagnosis for educational purpose, the point is that sometimes the cause of a disease can't be known until after death.

This book is an effort to probe a simpler understanding of disease from a biological perspective and show there can be simplicity underneath the apparent complexity. This book is about the nature of human diseases and my quest to understand human diseases from a systemic perspective.

As a medical doctor who is also a Biochemist, I want to explore the phenomenon of human disease and understand it from a more fundamental point of view and develop a unifying theory of human diseases. I want to go beyond the traditional approach of signs and symptoms of disease and their treatments. This is what doctors conventionally do. This is what medical students get taught in the medical school.

I want to look at human disease as a systemic disturbance to your body that endangers the continuation of the property of life.

I feel it is possible to apply system theory principles to human disease. The human body is a dynamic, self-regulating and adaptive complex system. A disturbance to the human body as a system is rectified by automated, regulatory mechanisms that will restore the system back to its optimal state in a manner typical of cybernetic systems. Physiologists call this the phenomenon of homeostasis. Any random deviation from the normalcy is met with a swift response to set deviation right. This dissipation of internal disruptions is characteristic of life systems, especially multi-cellular life systems.

The systems theory that emerged in the last few decades prefers to look at systems from a holistic view with less emphasis on the parts. The human body is a complex system that comprises of many interacting parts like organs, tissues and cells. We need to go above reductionist approaches to understand the human body in health and disease. The human body, like other multi-cellular life forms, are control systems amenable to descriptions according to the Cybernetic theory. There are several feedback loops based on information input operating to control the multiple components of the human body.

Cybernetics is almost synonymous with the system theory though there is a connotation of engineering systems when we talk about Cybernetics. No one can deny that our body has several engineering design principles in the organisation of our endocrine and nervous system. Cybernetics is the study of feedback control in a system that is based on communication. Its focus is on how the system processes the information, reacts to that information and changes the system in response. A whole lot of human function is precisely based on this type of information-based communication between body parts that act as control systems by their own right, often putting precision engineering to shame.

A typical aircraft has about 5,000-10,000 sensors that capture every detail of its operation. Effects of humidity, temperature and air pressure are assessed accurately. Individual parts of the aircraft are continuously monitored through sensors that emit warning signs predicting the failure of a part or a function much before the actual failure happens. This is no different from our human body showing distress or failure through clinical signs and symptoms. The doctors can pinpoint the source of the trouble based on the clinical sensors.

Our body consists of many sensors too. Their job is to continuously monitor all your vital functions 24/7 from the time you are born to the time you die. Just to mention a few examples, there is a sensor to detect falling energy levels in your body. We feel tired when our energy levels fall and start feeling hungry, but we do not how this happens. Inside your body, sensors detect falling glucose levels and send a signal to the 'feeding centre' in the brain to initiate a hunger response. That is when you start feeling grumpy and look for food to eat. Glucose molecules in food raise the blood concentration of glucose. At that time, the glucose sensor shuts itself off and stop sending SOS signals to the feeding centre.

This is pure Cybernetics.

Similar sensors exist throughout the body for several essential functions. Our body maintains constancy of many vital biochemical constituents like salt levels (sodium, potassium and chloride), gases (like oxygen and carbon dioxide), glucose, minerals (such as calcium, phosphorus, magnesium, iron and a host of others), water and nutrients. Their individual concentrations in the body fluctuate within a narrow range.

Remedial plans are kick-started to bring their levels back to normal whenever they deviate from the norm.

Some of these remedial actions are orchestrated by several regulatory mechanisms. These biochemical constituents are absolutely required to perform the function of life. They are not allowed to randomly deviate from an optimal concentration. When the optimal concentrations cannot be maintained, that is when problems start.

Water levels inside your body can fall due to various reasons like excessive sweating, heat loss of body secretions and so on. Your body gets dehydrated. This is no different from a drought. Information about body drought is picked up sensors in the brain. They dispatch signals to the 'thirst centre' in the brain to start the thirst response. Then we start feeling thirsty and drink fluids which help replenish the depleting fluids in the body. Once adequate amounts of fluid have been drunk, then the sensors send negative feedback to the thirst centre to switch it off. If it is not turned off by this negative feedback, there is a chance people will overdrink. Our body then faces the risk of flooding which is equally bad.

Your body heat is another cybernetic parameter. Body heat is controlled strictly like a thermostat in every sense of the word. What does a water heater do? It starts heating when the temperature falls below a set limit. It cools down when the temperature exceeds a limit. Our body works exactly like that.

Heat sensors in your body communicate to 'thermostatic' centre in the brain to achieve that. When our body heats up during fever, we take paracetamol tablets which acts by cooling this thermostatic centre in the brain. Fever itself is a response from our body to fight the microbes that have invaded our body. The higher temperature is deliberately induced by resetting the body thermostat to enable the killing of the microbe. Cold-blooded animals lack this thermostat mechanism and their body gets heated or cooled as per the prevailing environment. But warm-blooded animals like us have a thermostat in our body.

Our body has an efficient circulatory system. Blood is constantly pumped by the heart so there is a smooth flow of the blood throughout the body. When we have blood loss as in traumatic situations there is less blood volume inside our arteries. Sensors pick up the blood leak and immediately send 'cellular engineers' like platelets to seal the leak. A cascade of molecular reactions follows that literally prepare a 'sealant' to plug the leaking artery. All stops precisely after the job is done. It is amazing to know that the cells and molecules can perceive the 'plumbing' leak using sensors and initiate appropriate responses.

Our circulatory system needs the blood to be kept at an optimal pressure. There are pressure sensors located on arterial walls that can pick up falling blood pressure as well as rising blood pressures. Blood pressure control is a key self-regulatory function within our body. It cannot be too high or too low. If it is too low, then there is not enough blood circulating to reach the nook and corners of the body. It is like a drying river. Similarly, if the blood pressure becomes too high, there is a risk of the 'blood dam' breaching. This causes flooding within the cranium or abdominal cavity depends on where the breach happened. If the breach happens inside the brain that is what you call a stroke. Raised blood pressure, called hypertension, is one of the commonest medical problems faced by common man. Our own body has an extensive network of control mechanisms regulating blood pressure and keeping it within tolerable limits. I describe these mechanisms elsewhere in this book.

I can go on describing more and more such control units in our body an engineer would have devised in design of a human body. God indeed was the ultimate engineer who designed life systems! Physiologists would call such restorations of the constancy of the internal environment as 'Homeostasis'. An engineer would call it a cybernetic system. Both are the same. Spiritualists would call such restorations seen in our society in dire situations as the handy work of God, a miracle or even an avatar!

Many diseases make you suffer for a long time, and doctors call them chronic diseases. On the other hand, there are diseases that are killers. Death ensues in a very short time. What determines this? Are the chronic diseases an outcome of resetting the system (the body) to a different equilibrium set point? Can our body perform well at this altered set point well enough to allow continuation of the property of life? Can we assume that acute killer diseases disturb the system so much that it cannot function in a way compatible with life because the tolerance limits are exceeded in a short time?

The other intriguing argument I want to put forward is that

disease is a phenomenon that is unique to multi-cellular life forms. What is the reason behind my thinking? I feel this question has probably never been raised among biologists before. The question is: do unicellular life forms suffer from disease? Or is disease a truly a multi-cellular life property? There is no doubt that this is a fundamentally important question that needs an answer.

As I said before, I view diseases as a disorderly state. The disorder we refer to is the disorder prevailing amongst groups of cells. A single cell, or a small group of cells, does not face disorder, can it? For a disorder to arise, there must be many cells in the first place. Going back to the analogy of diseases as comparable to social maladies I do not think pre-historic man faced lot of social maladies back then.

He probably never knew civil unrest, illiteracy, economic inequalities, terrorism, etc. Because he lived in small social groups, there was little chance for social maladies to creep in. But the modern Homo sapiens who live in groups of millions of people living together is faced with all kinds of problems. That is why I can bet my last penny that unicellular life forms, like bacteria and viruses, will not suffer from anything like the disease phenomenon we see in multi-cellular life forms. I claim that the phenomenon of disease is peculiar to multi-cellular life forms like us. Animals, even other than man, do suffer from diseases as the veterinary doctors would acknowledge. But can we say the same for bacteria, fungi and viruses?

There must be a convincing argument for this bold claim that only multi-cellular life forms suffer from diseases. This intriguing biological characteristic needs proper explanation. My starting point for this argument is the assumption that a disease is a state of inter-cellular disorder.

How can we prove this? We need to delve into the nature of diseases.

Let us begin the journey.

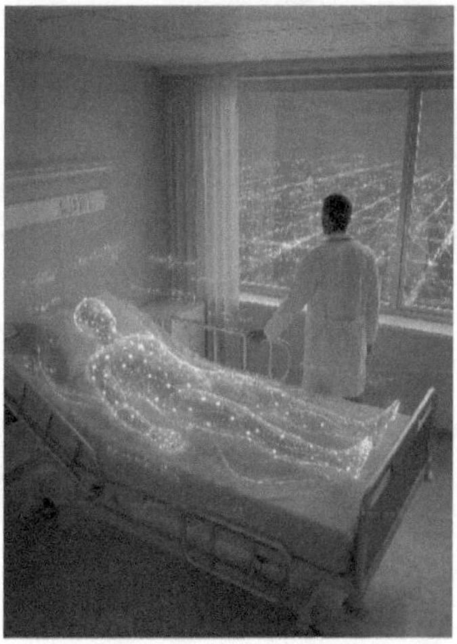

4. Defining the Term 'Disease'

JUST WHAT DO we mean by the term 'disease'? Can we define it? Most of us would define it as a pain, suffering, discomfort, disability and a potential forerunner to death. These definitions are descriptive. Apart from describing what the diseases are, do they really tell anything about the nature of disease?

Though we have come a long way towards understanding the molecular basis of most diseases, it is difficult to believe that there is still no satisfactory definition of the term 'disease'. This does not apply to the lay public only—doctors have the same difficulty. This lack of clear definition of disease and the hazy line of demarcation between 'disease' and 'non-disease' was highlighted in the survey conducted by the British Medical Journal (BMJ) in 2002. A huge list of conditions was thought of by health care professionals as indicative of diseases but were classified by BMJ as non-diseases.

The BMJ carried an article earlier in 1979, nearly 23 years prior to this 2002 survey, entitled *The Concept of Disease* emphasising the ambiguity in the meaning of the term. The authors suggested the name should refer to 'the sum of the abnormal phenomena displayed by a group of living organisms in association with a specified common characteristic, or a set of characteristics, by which they differ from the norm of their species in such as a way as to place them at a biological disadvantage'.

Unfortunately, this definition only describes the clinical features of the disease and in no way throws light on the underlying pathogenic mechanisms. This definition is inadequate for understanding disease because there is no mention of the reasons behind the abnormal phenomena that predispose the person to a biological disadvantage.

The World Health Organisation too has no definition of disease! Can you believe that? This is the organisation, headquartered in Geneva, which has a global role in conquest of human disease! WHO has only a definition for the term 'health' but not for disease. It defines health as 'a state of complete physical, mental and social well-being, and not merely the absence of disease and infirmity'. It is to be noted that there is no attempt to define disease here. Why is this? Is defining 'disease' so difficult that even WHO does not attempt it?

I looked up six leading textbooks of medicine, commonly used by medical students, but was dismayed to find that none of them defined disease. They describe all kinds of diseases, page after page, in several volumes big enough to be your pillow. But believe it or not, none of them defined the term 'disease'. I thought this was odd. It set me to think there is a need here. I am a medical doctor. I got on fine through all my years of medical education and practice until this point when I began to wonder about the nature of human diseases. Suddenly, it dawned on me that there is a need for a fresh thinking to develop a systemic understanding of human diseases.

A textbook of Pathology and a textbook of Biochemistry, both world leaders in the field of medical education, have a definition for the term 'disease'. The textbook of Pathology describes a disease process in terms of aetiology, pathogenesis and morphological changes in cells and organs and the functional consequences, which result in clinical symptoms. This is useful, but each disease will have its own description though it is possible to group the diseases based on the aetiology (such as nutritional diseases, genetic diseases, autoimmune diseases, inflammatory diseases, etc.).

It is also possible to classify the diseases by their cellular origin irrespective of their aetiology: into diseases of liver, kidneys, heart or nervous system etc. It is evident that the above approach to understand disease lacks an effort to find a common underlying basis of diseases that goes beyond the diverse aetiologies or the tissue of origin.

Harper's Textbook of Biochemistry defines disease as the result of "a perturbation of either the structures like DNA, or the amount of certain biomolecules, or important biochemical reactions and processes that operate to maintain the constancy of the internal cellular environment (regarding pH, osmolality, concentration of electrolytes). These perturbations are induced by many agents and often lead to severe alterations in the internal environment for which compensatory mechanisms can only operate for a finite period beyond which disease results".

This is the closest and the best definition I found yet for the term 'disease'! It views the human body as a system that can undergo disturbances that impairs the maintenance of stability of the system.

Harper's definition is attractive because it identifies a common underlying principle, viz. perturbation of the internal environment. But the deficiency of this approach is it fails to indicate a common proximate cause for the perturbation of the internal environment and how this perturbation causes the disease or death. In addition, there is no explanation for the variations in the duration of the disease processes (acute or chronic) nor does it indicate the critical factor(s) that determine why certain diseases lead to death while others do not, though they can drag on for years causing considerable morbidity.

In this book I explore the concept of disease from a biological perspective, viewing it as a failure to maintain the constancy of the internal environment of the body due to defects in intercellular communication. I show diverse disease-causing mechanisms produce convergent effects on key biochemical processes to bring about global disruption in the communication capabilities of the cells. I attempt to show that multi-cellular life systems like humans, consisting of trillions of cells, are vulnerable to cellular disorder as a result of this breakdown of information transfer resulting in an inability to function as a cohesive unit.

In summary, I claim that the information failure is the basis of cellular disorder associated with all human diseases.

Lay readers may struggle to understand what is meant by the term 'constancy of the internal environment'. Why does it matter? What does it mean? To explain this, let us look at a household. You have things in your house. Kitchen essentials like milk, coffee powder, tea bags, salt, sugar, cereals, bread, different types of vegetables, fruits, meat of various kinds and so on. As you consume these items the quantities of the items left at your home decreases. What do you do? You top up the items to restore the levels of the essential items to a level that will last for a period. To top up, you either go to the local grocery shop or to the supermarket or place an online order.

To top up these items you need the money. In order to get the money, you work. To do the work you maintain a car to travel to the site of work. You need fuel to run your car and you keep topping it up as in the case of groceries. Again, you need the money to buy the fuel. To get the money you work. Already we have seen that money has an indispensable role in keeping your nutrient levels constant in your kitchen as well as keeping your fuel levels constant in your car which, in turn, is needed to obtain the money to buy your groceries.

Money, or rather lack of it, has the potential to cause disruption to our lives. This could be a common factor in our domestic problems. One can trace much of our domestic problems to money. If we fix the money part, to a large extent we can fix our domestic problems.

What would happen if you ran out of milk? Probably nothing. You can still have a black coffee. What happens if you run out of coffee powder? You can go for your tea bags. What happens if you run out of tea bags? That is when you find that you cannot have a hot drink. What would happen if you cannot have a hot drink? You are not going to die, are you? We can extend this type of analysis to each of the items we discussed before.

At one point you will start noticing that some items like bread, rice, water, etc. are essential and you cannot function without them. You can live without coffee or tea but not without drinking water. Certainly not without energy-giving rice or wheat or bread, etc. These items will cause bigger impact on your life to the extent of disrupting your ability to function. You may run out of energy to do your household chores let alone do your office work.

In your body there are similar essential items like sodium, potassium (salts), glucose, amino acids, water, oxygen, etc. that are more important than others for continuation of life. There are several other minerals and vitamins etc. that are required for the bodily functions just like the optional food items that you may have in your kitchen. It could be some types of vegetables (replaceable by others) or fruits (replaceable by others) or cereals (replaceable by others) and so on. Some items like honey, sugar, biscuits, cakes, alcohol, etc. are dispensable in the sense you are not going to die without them. Lack of these items will not have an immediate impact but surely will disrupt orderly functions.

The body has several mechanisms to replenish the concentrations of the necessary ingredients and depending on the importance of the item, there are more restorative mechanisms in play. This is the equivalent of your grocery shopping. The list of items in the body that have life-sustaining potential include water, glucose, amino acids, sodium, potassium, calcium, magnesium, oxygen, etc. Any shortage of these items will lead to wider impact on bodily functions. They are like bread, rice, water, petrol, etc.

Therefore, the body evolved multiple mechanisms, often

redundant, so that there will be at least one or two ways of sourcing them when needed. These restorative mechanisms maintain the constancy of the internal bodily environment just like we top up items in our kitchen. There is a certain amount of time, depending on the importance of the item, where your kitchen can function—albeit with adjustments by family members. Beyond that, problems can start that might include hunger and starvation leading to nutritional deficiencies and consequent diseases.

The same thing happens inside the body. Homeostasis represents the term that encompasses all the remedial actions that are kick-started in the body that will restore the concentrations of the vital molecules. When the remedial mechanisms are unable to cope with the deviations of vital items then death ensues, or at least a lasting disease.

In summary, what matters is the availability of critically important molecules and entities inside the body that are needed by the body cells of all types. In real life I can think of at least three such items—fuel (food), oxygen (surprisingly applicable inside and outside our body) and water. Money is a man-made entity with the power to buy all you need for your inner and outer life. In that sense, absence of money can have far reaching consequences.

Going back to the definition of disease as an impairment of homeostatic mechanisms (i.e. mechanisms that will restore normalcy) the cause of this impairment is more likely to be lack of some entity that has a wider impact on bodily function. I suppose the same can be said of global problems too. Starvation (lack of glucose and amino acids) is a disease that afflicts human society as more than 50% of the world population goes to bed hungry.

Malnutrition has the same effect inside the human body as well as leading to a variety of diseases that might finally cause death. Fuel is another important requirement for our society to function without interruption. We are always looking for new types of fuels and one thing that can surely bring down the mighty Sapiens is a shortage of fuel. It will have the same effect as lack of oxygen that is the ultimate death-puller.

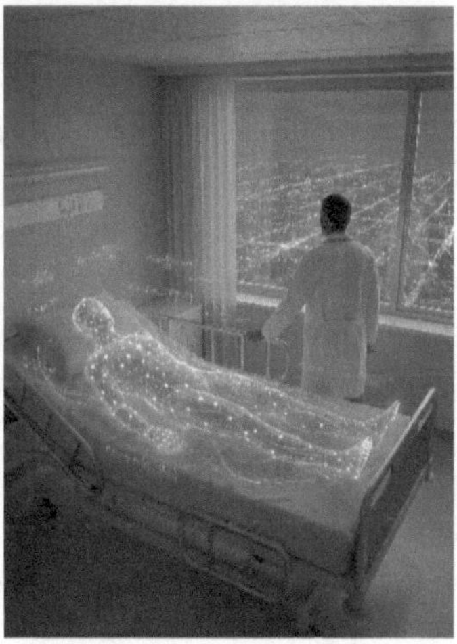

5. A Philosophical View of Diseases

DOCTORS ARE CONSIDERED next only to God. They are expected to perform miracles curing all diseases. They are expected to prevent death. Patients and their relatives have a great sense of gratitude to their doctors when all goes well. Many doctors become almost like family to their patients because the cured patient and their relatives do not easily forget the favour the doctor did for them.

Hospitals have evolved over time. Almost by default, people visit the hospital when something is awry with their body. I said before that this is no different from taking our car to the mechanic or taking the faulty machines and equipment to service centres. Depending on our knowledge and practice, we do a little bit of DIY with our cars and machines. Minor problems can be fixed if we have basic knowledge of design and function. Even if you are not medically trained, a little bit of self-cure is possible if you follow tips freely available from books and magazines. With regard to medical topics, the Internet is an easy source of information.

Hundreds of years ago, few were experts because we did not know much about human diseases. Shamans and village healers pretended to know about ailments and adopted treatments based on unscientific principles. But the poor people of the past had no way of knowing this and there was no other option anyway.

Similarly, if you are a member of a native tribe living a jungle or on a mountain, you will not have the luxury of a doctor or a hospital. You might only have the services of a community member who pretends to be a healer. This is the case in many rural parts of the world even today where villagers still lack proper healthcare.

Self-help is possible even today for some minor illnesses. You do not need a doctor for it. But once things look serious, we run to the hospital. Quite often patients who are in their end stage of their lives, due to some sort of serious illnesses such as advanced cancers or major traumatic injuries, are taken to the hospitals in their dying moments almost as if it is the right thing to do and probably the only thing to do. That is proper if there is hope, but, in many cases, there is none, but you do not want to accept it. People look at rushing to the hospital as natural because that is where the doctors are, and they are Gods.

Rushing to hospital in an emergency, sometimes even for a non-emergency, is a widespread human behaviour. Most people end up in the hospital if they survive those precious few minutes needed for their transportation. There is big hope in their minds that some miracle will happen. There does not seem to be any other option really in their minds. That is why even a dying patient is rushed to the hospital—almost as a ritual. When death comes it feels somehow right that it happened in a hospital. Even when death was inevitable people prefer to die in a hospital. This may be because of the slim hope that some miracle can happen due to an ingenious nurse or doctor.

Cancer hospitals in many parts of the world seem to have the view that it is futile to keep some of the terminally ill cancer patients in their wards. Many a time, dying patients, such as those with terminal cancer, are sent home to die in peace. Dying in such circumstances at their own homes amid their loved ones, might even be considered dignified. But this is a rarity. In many hospitals these days there is a 'Do not resuscitate' policy in effect. What this policy means is that dying patients, who have chronic, incurable conditions, will not receive any attempts to be resuscitated if they suffered a cardio-respiratory arrest. This is because—even if they are temporarily brought back to life—their pre-existing conditions will prevent them from surviving much longer. Then what is the point of calling the Emergency teams? These teams usually consist of anaesthetists, emergency room doctors, cardiologists, nurses, etc. and they must rush literally in seconds to the site of the emergency call leaving behind what they have been doing at the time of the Code Blue call. It is a waste of time to focus on hopeless patients; these valuable resources can be directed at patients who have a chance.

In a way, people living primitive life in remote parts of the world are probably less afraid of death than people living in advanced societies. Diseases are not feared simply because they do not know about them. Primitive man living thousands of years ago had no clue about diseases. They were not, therefore, worried about the consequence of the diseases.

Today we worry about heart attacks, cancer, obesity, diabetes, arthritis and a whole range of other diseases. Even lay press covers a lot of articles on such diseases and people worry about them. Many spend time worrying about the chances they might get those diseases. The ones who got them worry about the cost of the treatment and the disruption in their personal lives. Those with the advanced diseases know the eventual outcome and start worrying about the impending death.

The recent Corona virus pandemic is a stark example of how mankind can be terrorized by the fear of a disease.

Primitive people of the past had no such worries because they had no idea about the diseases and there was nothing they had to fear about. Disease and death are viewed as destiny by primitive people. They accept death as something unavoidable. There are no institutionalised preparations for the inevitable death. Death is accepted as normal and may even be viewed as God's punishment. There is little need for elaborate pre-death dramas. The structure of their simple societies offers little scope for them anyway. If you do not have a hospital or a doctor, where would you rush them to?

The fear of death is probably correlated to the complexity of the societies. In a highly complex modern society, people have too many strings attached to their personal lives. If someone is about to die or has serious disease that will affect the ability to work, there are more worries about the implications to the family from a financial point of view. Who will pay the mortgage, the credit card companies, and educational expenses for the children, food for the surviving family, etc.?

These worries come to the forefront in our minds when we face death or disease. Our society is structured in such a way that earning a salary is like breathing oxygen. When you are about to die or get incapacitated due to crippling disease, the primary worry is the cessation of earning and the effect it has on the lives of the family members. This leads to frantic efforts to prevent the inevitable death, like rushing to the hospital in blind faith.

What does this discussion above in the last few paragraphs mean? Does it mean it is wrong to access healthcare in an institution if you suffer from a disease? Probably no, but what is wrong is the over expectation from the public about what the medical community can do for you.

Not only we have come to expect the miracles from doctors and hospitals, but we have gone one step further in the wrong direction. We have now learned to blame the doctor and the hospital for perceived failures to reverse the course of the disease and death. This is a worrying development in our society over the last 40-50 years. People realised that someone can be held responsible for their diseases and death. The doctor is expected by default to know about your disease and the way to treat it. If the doctor fails to make the diagnosis or there is a delay in the diagnosis resulting in morbidity or mortality, then the doctor is at fault and not you who had the 'faulty' body. The hospital also is held accountable. Many patients, or their relatives, have earned fortunes from their illnesses.

Only in the 20th century did diseases become money-spinners. Diseases may lower survival fitness in Darwinian terms but the evolution of healthcare in the modern world led to a curious situation whereby patients can exploit the weakness to their own advantage.

Going back to the point I raised a little while ago as to why people almost always ritually take the diseased and dying to the treatment centres, I guess this is because this concept is so much entrenched in their minds that they have started believing that access to healthcare is their birth right. The government is seen to be ultimately responsible for providing care for the diseased. In many countries like the US, there is no free health care. The insurance companies took on this role as sponsors of the health care delivery, but the patient pays the premium. Because you have paid for it you expect good service in return.

Of course, doctors do a great job in majority of the cases but, due to various factors, sometimes things go wrong. Mistakes happen. Wrong diagnosis could be made, or theew could be delays in making the diagnosis. This may be because of the limitations of the hospital as an organisation. For a person who walks in with headache, the doctor cannot simply order a CT scan to rule out a brain tumour. They must rationalise their thinking and go for the simple Paracetamol first. Then look at signs and symptoms and response to initial treatment.

At some stage the doctor may think about more serious causes of the headache if the symptom persists for a long time or recurs often. The doctor tries to prioritise more expensive investigations for patients who need them most. An insurance company will not approve a CT scan of the head for everybody with headache. This is only an example. This applies to a lot of other disease conditions where a doctor must work like a detective trying to look at the obvious and more common conditions before thinking about rare possibilities. Apart from resource availability within the hospital to do CT scans and MRI scans for everybody, there may be external pressures from insurance companies. So, availability of modern technology is one thing, but using it indiscreetly is another.

Man has been troubled by diseases since ancient times. Our understanding of diseases has grown incredibly in the last century and we have come a long way from treating diseases by magic and prayer.

Ancient man was convinced that disease was divine punishment and therefore a mark of sin. This conviction was quite widespread in the ancient world. This belief was passed on by the Mesopotamian cultures to the biblical Hebrews, which continued well into the Christian Medieval Europe.

Greeks believed that Gods could bring an illness or widespread pestilence, which needed prayer, sacrifice or purification to appease the offended God. The Egyptians considered symptoms like cough, fever, swelling and skin rash as individual diseases and there was very little effort to group the symptoms into categories. The ancient Chinese regarded disease not so much a result of punishment for sin but the inevitable result of acting contrary to 'Tao', the universal principle. Illnesses could also be caused by forces beyond one's control, like wind and atmospheric conditions, which upset the harmonious inner balance of 'Yang' and 'Yin'.

For a very long time in human history, diseases were thought to be due to evil spirits. This was believed to happen when some wrong was committed by the diseased man and disease was viewed as a punishment. The remedy was in setting right the wrong he had done or in appeasing God through the doctor or shamanistic rituals. That is why practitioners of medicine have always been held in high regard in our society. It is very common for modern doctors to be treated with respect in many parts of the world and are often considered next only to God.

Primitive man was no different. For him the witch doctor was the agency through which he can establish contact with God and seek help. Primitive societies—even to date—continue to have such 'medicine men' that lack formal training and often have no knowledge of diseases, but are sought for treatment simply out of belief or tradition. These village healers are usually priests in the local temples and/or shamans.

Expelling the evil spirit was required as treatment and this required help. In the pre-historic past, and in fact until very recent history, the help was sought through prayer or magic. Expulsion of so-called evil spirit by rituals is practiced even today in rural parts of the world. Shamanism refers to the primitive practice of healing through the agency of a healer, often a village priest. The process of curing of diseases was believed to be achieved by mending the soul. Shamans were thought to be intermediaries to the spirit world and solutions to human problems, including diseases, were sought from the spirits. The shaman tries to cure diseases by gifting, threatening, flattering or wrestling the disease-spirit. Shamanism is based on the belief that invisible forces or spirits affect the lives of people by unwanted entry into the visible world.

Diseases were thought to be caused by factors in the spiritual realm and someone needed to enter the spirit world to set them right. Shamans were the ones expected to do it. They did that by 'entering' supernatural realms or dimensions. Guidance was sought from the other worlds for problems, including diseases. Shamans were able to make people believe that they are in a different world by modifying the consciousness, either auto-hypnotically or using entheogens. Entheogenic substances used included those that were derived from plants and fungi like Psilocybin mushrooms, Cannabis, Tobacco, Fly agaric, Deadly nightshade, Datura, San Pedro cactus, Morning glory, Hawaiian Baby Wood rose, Salvia divinorum, etc. Extracts of these plants had substances that make the user go into a trance or into some form of altered consciousness.

Shamans across different cultures also used many other methods of inducing beliefs in susceptible people. Drumbeating is used by shamans by Inuit in Siberia and in many other cultures.

Drumbeating is a widely used practice across ancient cultures for achieving an altered state of consciousness. It was supposed that this altered state of consciousness will allow travel between the real world and the spiritual world.

In many North and South American cultures and in Asia feathers are used in healing rituals. The reason was that birds were believed to be messengers of spirits because they could fly in space. Smoking various tobaccos and psychoactive herbs like cannabis is used in shamanistic practices. Sadhus in India use Cannabis and shamans in Americas are known to use tobacco in a ritualistic setting. Swords are used in some cultures as a protection for the shaman from evil spirits when he wanders in the spirit world.

Shamans still exist even today. They are seen primarily in indigenous cultures living in jungles, tundra, deserts and rural villages in the modern civilisation. I have seen this practiced even today by village priests in South India by so-called priests who attempt to drive the evil spirit out of the mind of the psychotic patient. They beat the patients with Neem leaves repeatedly and harshly, uttering 'magic' words, and they threaten the spirit with bad consequences if it failed to leave. One could say that shamans are prevalent even today in the parts of the world where there are many illiterate people and/or places where there is no access to modern medical care.

The difficulty in treating mental illnesses, even in modern times and even with all the advances in medicine, is evident. For many mental illnesses, the aetiology is unclear and the treatment is so non-specific that it affects non-targeted parts of the brain.

Imagine what would have been the case in the distant past.

Without knowledge about the body organs, immune systems, microbes and our physiology, what do you expect primitive man to do? Modern medicine only started developing from about 18th and 19th century and has made rapid progress in the 20th century, but diseases were prevalent since the origin of man hundreds of thousands of years ago.

A lot of diseases man suffers from now are now known to be

due to the life-style changes, like inactivity, excess fat or sugar intake, stress, etc. but they are only a minority of illnesses afflicting man. There are many diseases that occur in man due to genetic mutations and susceptibility, infectious agents, nutritional lack, cancer and mental illnesses which may have bothered man since time immemorial.

Egyptians were great healers. Ancient papyri texts that survived tell us that Egyptians had a good knowledge of medicinal herbs as well as repair of physical injuries. I suppose the healing and repair of physical wounds is more relevant in the ancient Egyptian society because of their long tradition of building massive monuments and the more than likely event of frequent physical harm to the workers. They had a system of sick leave and early retirement in case of injury to workers. Egyptian labourers were fed a diet rich in radish, onion and garlic which are now known to be rich in natural antibiotics like allicin, allistatin and raphanin.

This must have helped to contain outbreaks of diseases in crowded labour camps. Powdered liver, rich in Vitamin A, was given by Egyptians to cure night blindness! Honey was used an antiseptic by Egyptians to treat wounds. This ancient cure has been adopted by even the British military to treat soldiers who suffered burns. A study comparing the efficacy of honey and sulfadiazine in dressing the burn victims showed the honey was far more effective. This is attributed to the antioxidant and anti-microbial properties of honey.

A concoction made from the Willow tree was used to treat toothache. It is now known the Willow bark is the basis of modern aspirin. Parasitic diseases have afflicted Egyptians of the past and present. The ancient Egyptians used pomegranate (known to contain high levels of Tannin capable of paralyzing parasitic worms) to expel parasites.

It can be surmised that much of the medical knowledge possessed by the ancient Egyptians about human body and illnesses were derived from their practice of embalming the dead which required them to anatomically dissect the body. This gave them a good idea of organ functions—at least which organ was responsible for what.

Greeks believed that most human ailments could be cured by praying to the God of Medicine, Asclepius. They built temples called Aesclepions where Greeks went to heal. Hippocrates changed the way Greeks saw the diseases. In fact, Hippocrates laid the foundation for Modern Medicine by separating medicine from divine. He initiated the practice of looking for symptoms and physical examination and obtaining a history from the patients. Modern day doctors still do them—which speak of the enormous contribution made by Hippocrates to the medical sciences. The Hippocratic Oath is still undertaken by doctors when they embark on a career of medical healing.

Some medical appliances like scissors, forceps and catheters used by the Greeks in the olden days are still recognizable in a modern-day surgical theatre. Greeks thought of human diseases as an imbalance in one of the four humours—Sanguine, Choleric, Melancholic and Phlegmatic. Diet, age, climate, etc. affected these humours and led to the diseases. In one sense, we now consider this as comparable to perturbations in our internal environment which need to be rectified.

Till well into the Middle Ages, the Greeks treated their diseases by trying to balance the humours. Greeks believed in a Goddess of hygiene called Hygeia. Hygeia was supposed to the daughter of Asclepius, the God of Medicine and healing. Along with these Gods, they also worshipped Panacea (God of universal remedy) and Apollo (God of Music, Healing and Prophecy) who are all mentioned in the Hippocratic Oath recited even today. So, it can be safely assumed that even Hippocrates did not totally abandon a role for the healing Gods in the treatment of human diseases.

Romans placed more emphasis on cleanliness in preventing diseases. They knew that dirt and poor hygiene were somehow linked to human diseases: not very far from the modern truth. They built aqueducts to supply clean water to the citizens. Roman engineers built massive public baths to help their people clean themselves and prevent diseases. Roman baths can be seen in many places even today. In England, there is a massive Roman bath that can be seen in the city of Bath. I visited it a couple of times. It was apparently built almost 2,500 years ago, and it is unbelievably impressive.

Though medicine has evolved over the millennia, there are still ancient medical practices that have survived suggesting that the ancient people managed to understand the nature of some human diseases better. Acupuncture, developed by the Chinese around 2,000-2,500 years ago, is still widely in use across the world. Though it is removed from the modern theories of physiology and anatomy, the wide uptake of this art of medicine indicates the possibility that the Chinese probably deciphered the nature of many diseases in their own way. How placing needles on designated pressure points helps not only in treatment of pain but even other diseases is not known.

Craniotomy means opening the skull. This practice has been used since pre-historic times—even during the stone-age. Archaeologists unearthed skulls with circular holes showing people did this as part of some treatment. It is believed that pre-historic people attempted to open the skull to drive away evil spirits which they thought were responsible for epilepsy or mental illnesses. But the striking truth is that craniotomies are even today used as a standard neurosurgery procedure for management of brain tumours, hematomas and skull fractures.

Hippocrates described the procedure of cauterization (burning) of a part of the body using heat for treatment of some conditions. Cauterization is still used today to cut tissue or to stop bleeding. Even procedures like caesarean sections and tracheostomy were practiced by Romans and Greeks—which is amazing.

History tells us that humanity has suffered from disease outbreaks that had major impact on the society and the course of the human history. Often, the population dwindled following major epidemics. Death of tens and hundreds of thousands of people left the society in shatters.

Greek history has an account of a disease epidemic that happened around 430-426 BC. This is now believed to be a devastating plague, which some believe to have been typhoid fever. This disease is thought to have killed one third of the population of Athens, including their leader Pericles. This is one instance demonstrating a big change in the course of history due to a microbial culprit. Pericles had dominated this part of the world around this time, and it was said to be a golden period. All this came to a halt due to the fact he died because of a disease that killed him and tens of thousands of his citizens.

The balance of power shifted from Athens to Sparta. A historian called Thucydides who lived during this disease, also contracted it, but he survived to write about the plague. Based on his writings, modern academics and medical scientists consider epidemic typhus the most likely cause of this outbreak.

Another historical epidemic was seen in the English colony of Jamestown, Virginia where almost entire population was wiped out from this small town due to typhoid. Typhoid fever killed more than 6,000 settlers between 1607 and 1624. 81,360 Union soldiers died of typhoid or dysentery during the American Civil War. As recently as the late 19th century, typhoid fever mortality averaged 65 per 100,000 people a year.

This became even worse when the typhoid death rate was 174 per 100,000 people in 1891. Public sanitation conditions were poor during these times with rising populations. The industrial revolution that began early in the 19th century was beginning to cause an explosion in population, but the consequence of crowding led to challenges in sanitation.

A carrier of a disease in the society was easily able to transmit the disease to many others. The most notorious carrier of typhoid fever known in medical history, was Mary Mallon, also known as Typhoid Mary. She became the first American carrier to be identified and traced back in 1907. Her profession was cooking which, unfortunately, was ideal for spreading Typhoid. She spread the disease until the authorities tracked the source of the infection to her. She was made to quit cooking, but she cheated the authorities and returned to her profession under a false name. Finally, she was kept under quarantine for over 26 years.

Recent corona virus pandemic is one such major event in human history. It has led to unprecedented steps that we never dreamt of. Entire countries were shut down to stop spreading the disease.

Modern medicine gave rise to unrealistic hopes in the past couple of decades. We started believing every medical condition should be treatable and manageable. There are many diseases we can hardly do anything about. Despite the incredible advances in medical sciences over the last century the concept of disease is still poorly understood.

Surprisingly, as I told you before, there is a lack of agreement about what constitutes a disease and there has been very little effort to find a unified understanding of human disease. Medical knowledge exploded in the last few decades to the extent that medical practice is increasingly becoming super-specialised. Doctors drown themselves in endless detail about various diseases of diverse organ systems and there is hardly any attempt to synthesise a unifying view of the phenomenon of disease.

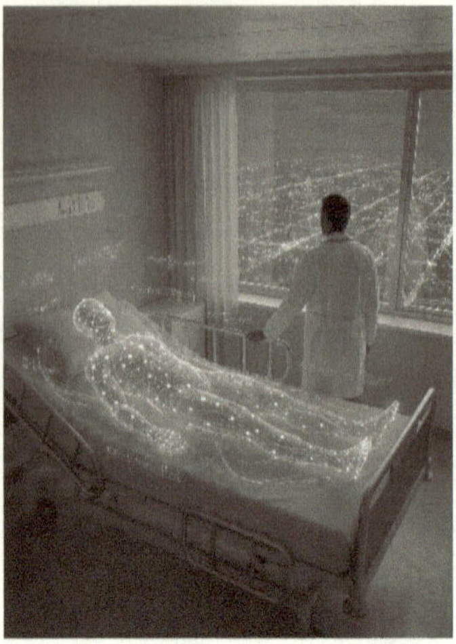

6. Curing Diseases Seems to be an Animal Instinct

IS DISEASE AN exclusively human phenomenon? The answer is absolutely no. Even animals fall sick. That is why we have vets. For that matter, even plants can become ill. All multi-cellular life forms are to disease. Even aliens, if they are multi-cellular, will not escape from disease.

Unicellular life forms like the bacteria can get infected by viruses called bacteriophages. These bacteriophages can infect a bacterial cell and hijack the host to utilize the cell's machinery to make copies of the phage that will burst out at one stage by killing the bacteria or live inside the bacterial host in a symbiotic way—making more copies as the bacteria divides.

Let us now focus on how wild animals treat themselves when they fall sick. In domesticated animals of course we have vets who do that. What about animals living in the wild? The fact that animals seek medicinal plants when needed suggests healing could be a biological trait. There is no need to think that we are special in that we have 'invented' medical sciences.

To be precise, man relies on plants and fungi heavily for medicines. It is no secret that more than half of medicines used by us in the practice of modern medicine are plant products or are made by lowly fungi. The antibiotics we use to treat bacterial diseases are really chemicals made by the fungi in self-defence to beat the same bacteria that we are trying to treat!

The first antibiotic Penicillin, which Alexander Fleming discovered, is made by a fungus. The anti-malarial drug Artemisinin (or Qinghaosu) is derived from a Chinese medicinal herb Artemisia annua. The other commonly used malaria drug called Chloroquine is a fully synthetic analogue of quinine, the natural alkaloid derived from Cinchona shrubs.

Many anti-cancer medicines we use are plant-derived too! Just as nature has evolved food for life systems, we also see the bountiful medicines too! The formulary of Mother Nature is obviously not for sole human use. Other life systems also use the same formulary. Unlike us the animals don't have to pay. It is the mankind who has created this system of 'manufactured' medicines that cost a fortune.

It is an interesting point to discuss why nature evolved medicinal substances. One could surmise that they exist to restore order and balance in life systems. Many of these medicinal substances may be made by plants, shrubs and microbes for their own needs including defence but one cannot discount the theory that they are there to help maintain orderly function in multicellular life systems.

Plants are the groceries or supermarkets that Nature created in a non-profitable sense where life systems can 'shop' for their food and medicines. Plants give us fruits and vegetables so that life systems can obtain a supply of essential molecules to run their life processes and what do the plants get back? Dispersal of their seeds for propagation of their species. In the same way, we need to think of medicinal substances as incentives nature gives us to make our lives better.

If you want to ask the question, why should Nature do that for us? Try to first answer the question—'why should Nature give us food?'

The observation of animals eating foods not part of their usual diet, has led to the belief that animals self-medicate themselves with natural remedies found in leaves, roots, seeds and rock minerals. This has been referred to as Zoo pharmacognosy.

African elephants, when they are pregnant and nearing their term, have been observed to seek out a shrub (a member of the borage family) that grew in areas even far away from their shelter. The leaves and bark of this tree are chewed by the elephants and a few days later they give birth. It appears that the elephants seek a natural remedy to induce themselves into labour. It is very interesting that Kenyan women are known to use the same plant to make a labour-inducing tea!!

Chimps have been observed to roll up the prickly Aspilla shrubs and then swallow them. They are also known to peel the stems and eat the pith of Vernonia plant. It is interesting that Tanzanian folk medicine includes both Vernonia and Aspilla for stomach upsets and fevers. These plants have been studied to have anti-microbial properties and anti-parasitic effects.

Baboons in Ethiopia living near the Awash waterfalls have learnt to use some medicinal property of the tree Balanite aegyptica (Desert date). What is intriguing is that only baboons living below the waterfalls ate the tree's fruit and not those baboons who live above the waterfalls. The reason is the balanite fruit has the property of repelling a parasitic worm found inside the water snails in this area. When the baboons eat the water snails, they get infected with the parasites. Those baboons living above the waterfalls do not encounter these water snails and therefore are not affected by these parasites. Therefore, these baboons do not touch balanite fruits.

Colobus monkeys living on the island of Zanzibar steal and eat the charcoal from the bonfires made by the people living here. The reason is hard to believe. They act like toxicologists. By eating the charcoal, they are doing exactly what hospitals do to treat poison victims. Charcoal has the property of adsorbing toxic chemicals. The Colobus monkey is trying to counteract the toxic phenols contained in the mangos and almond that grow there. Can you believe that?

Even some birds like the South American parrot and macaw can get rid of toxic compounds in the diet by adopting similar approaches. They eat solids with a high kaolin content to rid themselves of poisons like cyanide contained in the fruit seeds they eat. Kaolin has been used for centuries in different cultures for treatment of stomach and intestinal upsets. Kaolin is also a standard content in some modern medicine formulations used for intestinal complaints.

In Northern California dusky-footed rats bring fresh bay leaves into their sleeping nests to control an abundance of fleas. Studies have shown that the bay leave extracts worked with as much as 80% comparable efficiency as a powerful chemical repellent called Diethyl Toluamide sold in the shops.

Avoiding parasites and pathogens is something animals do and they have a variety of ploys to achieve this objective. Avoiding grazing on forage adjacent to recently dropped faeces has been documented in sheep, horses and cattle. Felids and canids practice den sanitation. One aspect of the feeding behaviour of carnivores and omnivores is the risk of getting infected when they eat the dead carcass of some animal that has probably even died of an infectious disease or has been dead for a long time and therefore grew microbes. Because pathogens are species-specific, this cross-infection does not happen. It turns out that animals will never eat the dead carcass of a dead animal of a conspecific which has been referred to as cannibalism taboo. Perhaps this can be said to be true of even human who never eat other humans. We humans may have stumbled upon the idea of frying or baking their meats in order to get rid of the pathogens!! The taste that followed this fire-induced grilling was only an added, perhaps, an unexpected bonus.

Avoidance of pathogens by quarantine may be thought to be a practice adopted by humans especially in national borders like what we did for containing the corona virus epidemic. Even animals tend to do that. Repulsion of strange conspecifics has been seen practiced by primates. Rodents cannibalize sick infants to protect the littermates.

Animals are well known to lick their wounds to help in the healing process. It is well known that saliva contains several anti-microbial and wound-healing substances—including lactoferrin, lysozyme, epidermal growth factors etc. Laboratory experiments demonstrated that dog saliva can prevent the growth of E. coli and S. Canis which are two most common organisms that cause wound contamination in animals. Male rats compulsively lick the penis after copulation. Rat saliva has been shown to be effective in warding off bacteria that can cause genital infections.

Grooming as a ploy to remove ectoparasites like ticks, fleas and lice is well known in the animal kingdom. Several studies have shown this in ungulates, mice, cats. Animals also resort to fly-repelling behaviours like ear twitching, head-tossing, leg stamping, muscle-twitching, etc.

It can be safely said that many types of behaviours are used by animals to control their diseases. Avoidance of pathogens, avoidance of parasites, intake of medicinal plants, quarantine, caring for the sick, sexual selection of partners endowed with disease-resistant genes, and even controlled exposure to pathogens to potentiate the immune system are some of those types of behaviours. The mothers of some early maturing species tend to pass on the infant around to group members to expose the infant to pathogens in a limited way. Species that have a long maturation stage do not show this behaviour. Weanling young of carnivores are sensitized to microbes as the mother brings the kill dragging it over dirt and filth.

Ultimately, these diverse animal behaviours clearly point to one thing. All life forms have one major goal—to preserve their lives. Pathogens and parasites are impediments to their continued existence and animals want to get rid of them no different from humans. Why do these pathogens pose a threat to the life of the animals infected? How do they make the animals sick and diseased? Infections and infestations in other animal species have the same ill-effects as seen in humans.

Basically, microbes are life systems by their own right. They seek nutrients to survive. They seek a place to survive in nature. For both these reasons they forcefully and slyly gain unlawful entry into other life systems.

This is medically termed an infection.

Given the number of diverse microbes, there are innumerable types of infections suffered by animals including humans. The microbes target different organs in their host animals. Their entry into the host disturbs the dynamics of the host survival. There may be effects on certain key processes that help maintain the constancy of the internal environment of the host. When this happens there is by my definition a disease. Outright death of the host animal may not be good for the invading microbial life system.

Evolutionarily, microbes and animals have sought balance. Some microbes do not cause debilitating or life-threatening disturbance to the host internal environment whereas there are other microbes which cause far more destruction or death. They attack vital organs like the lungs, heart or brain and kill. SARS-Corona virus, for example, targets the lung to cause pneumonia. There are so many other pathogens which can target the same lungs causing the same pneumonia disease. It is for the doctor to figure out the culprit.

In the same way, the polio virus targets the nervous system while the brain fever virus will target the brain. Pathogens usually only attack one type of organ.

In simple words, infections are a battle between life systems for nutrients and survival. That is why animals evolve mechanisms to ward off the microbes. I suppose infectious diseases are representative of colonial tendencies that we have seen throughout history. Microbes colonise foreign lands i.e., bodies of life systems.

They declare war with us.

The infections that ensue are vigorously fought back by man

and other life systems.

Who wins the battle?

With the aid of medical technology, we win a significant number of these battles, but we encounter epidemics like the recent COVID that shake us up. As of now we are yet to recover from the jolt given by this invisible enemy. We will need another decade to recoup the losses the world over.

COVID was truly a World War III. Usually, man is known to kill his own kind in wars. On this occasion this World War III was initiated by the Corona virus and, for once, man was seen to cooperate with each other in fighting the COVID war.

It was the Corona virus versus the allies—all the nations in the world collectively on one side which is rather unusual. A lowly microbe managed to unite the world. As per Hollywood film makers—only an alien invasion would have such a unifying effect on humanity.

Here we saw this happen thanks to a virus.

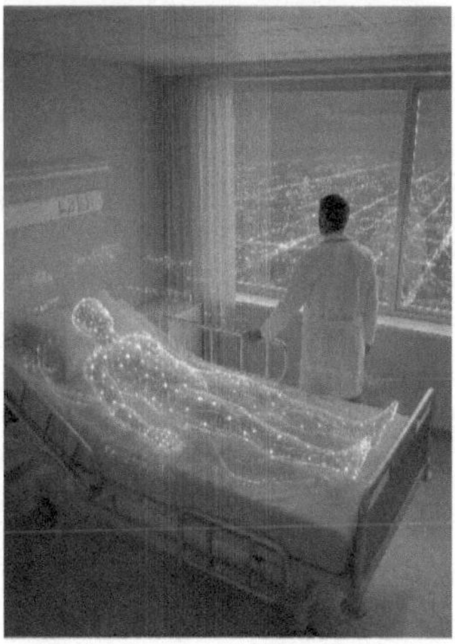

7. How do Doctors Diagnose a Disease? The Inside Detective

DOCTORS ARE OFTEN criticized for taking a "shotgun" approach—ordering every possible diagnostic test without aligning them to the patient's specific signs and symptoms. Instead, medicine requires a more disciplined, detective-like method. Using the available evidence—clinical signs, symptoms, and patient history—the physician works to identify the underlying cause of disease. This cause could be anything from an infection to a toxin to cancer. The process involves systematically narrowing possibilities and ruling out potential causes based on the evidence at hand.

The evidence includes mainly the symptom the patient has told him. He or she supplements this evidence by doing a physical examination where he looks for physical manifestations of the disease.

Doctors call this the 'sign'.

A 'sign' differs from a 'symptom' in medical parlance. A 'sign' is some external manifestation of the disease which the doctor found by a specific observational act during a physical examination of the patient. This is like the detective examining the scene of the crime. Whereas a 'symptom' is one which the patient feels for himself—like a pain, vomiting, fever etc. Usually a 'symptom' is what the patient tells the doctor about the reason why he visited the doctor. This is called the presenting complaint in medical parlance again. Symptoms told by the patient and the signs elicited by the doctor tell a lot usually. These are like circumstantial evidence collected at the scene of the crime. In many cases it is like an open and shut case. There is a clear idea in the mind of the doctor what the problem is that is bothering the patient. In such cases he can already think about a treatment plan. At least, he can start thinking of treating the 'symptom'.

Symptomatic treatment refers to the attempt made by the doctor to relieve the 'symptom' by simple remedies to buy some time. A patient coming with pain anywhere in the body will thank the doctor if he or she can relieve the pain first. The underlying, root cause of the pain needs to be worked out later. The doctor will rely on some diagnostic tests to do that. This is like the detective sending for some tests to the crime lab. Once the cause is found then the doctor will work on a more definitive, long-lasting treatment aiming for a cure. It may take time and more diagnostic investigations.

Results of diagnostic tests add more weight towards presence or absence of disease. The purpose of a diagnostic test can be broadly two-fold. Either the doctor is interested in knowing the presence or absence of a diagnostic condition. Or he is interested in finding the offending culprit that caused the disease. In the case of the latter scenario the doctor knows the presence of the disease but is interested in finding the cause. In both scenarios a positive and negative result in a diagnostic test tells a doctor something.

He eliminates the offending culprit one by one.

In an emergency there is a justifiable need to do many diagnostic tests simultaneously to save time. For non-emergency conditions this luxury is not there. The patient unfortunately thinks different. The patient thinks that, in the 21st century, with all the exciting medical advances, it should be easy to make the diagnosis.

The modern patient is spoiled and has high expectations.

Many family practitioners in their clinics see patients who have minor symptoms. The patients with major symptoms, or emergency conditions, go to the hospital emergency department directly. For the family practitioner who sees only the non-emergency patients he must consider common causes first while trying to make a diagnosis on a patient who is otherwise well. The patient may be somebody who is visiting the doctor straight from work or home, having done their usual chores. The doctor cannot afford to think of investigating rare medical conditions for everyone who has just walked into his clinic while being able to carry about out his or her usual life.

Moreover, for low-incidence rare conditions results of diagnostic tests can give misleading answers. In some diseases making a false-positive diagnosis is as harmful as having a false-negative diagnosis. All tests have a certain degree of false-positive and false negative rate. If the disease condition was a rare one this will have an impact on the false positive and false negative rate of the diagnostic test. The likelihood of a person having a disease due to an offending agent increases with increasing evidence. The increasing evidence can be in the form of a test result from a second or third diagnostic test. The combined evidence adds weight to the possibility that the patient really has the disease or that it is due to a particular causative agent. This is Bayesian probability.

It is almost no different from our perception about people.

If someone did something wrong, our perception about that person will depend on whether he or she has done the same thing before. If yes, then we say 'Oh, yeah, that's a troublemaker'.

Inwardly, we have done a Bayesian probability assessment in our minds. We assess the pre-event probability whether the guy is a troublemaker based on his past behaviour. The likelihood that he is a troublemaker increases with the history. In the court a convict gets sentenced based on the weight of all evidence combined. Fingerprints, witnesses, blood stains, CCTV footage etc. all adds up to the probability that a person accused really committed the crime.

With less of the evidence available there is little possibility to pin the murder on the accused and he gets the benefit of doubt and the jury let him go. Similarly, it is true that some types of evidence from the crime scene may be misleading or inaccurate or even wrong. The wrong guy gets punished. There is a saying that the justice system works on the principle that all are innocent until proven guilty.

Our justice system also works to uphold another laudable principle—the innocent should never get punished though an occasional guilty can escape.

Many diagnostic tests are like this.

They produce results that may have inherent uncertainties due to the analytical procedure or variations in the patient. The evidence produced by lab diagnostic results can be inconclusive or, even worse, point in the wrong direction. It can be false-positive or false-negative. That means the innocent gets punished and the guilty are escaping!

Therefore, doctors combine the weight of clinical signs and symptoms to the diagnostic test result in order to make an interpretation before making that final judgement—the diagnosis. It is quite possible that the doctors make a wrong diagnosis in a certain number of patients due to misleading diagnostic reports or they are duped by symptoms and signs which are non-specific. It is not unknown that the court of law sometimes hands out punishment to the innocent.

The other implication is that once a diagnosis is made, rightly or wrongly, it remains in the medical records of the patient probably for a long time before it is disproved and removed. This is I suppose like a person getting a criminal record when he or she is wrongfully or rightfully convicted. Even otherwise the patient carries the stigma of 'being diseased', especially a disease that has undesirable features like mental illnesses. This stigma may even last the lifetime of the person concerned.

In the case of some high-profile diseases like HIV, which is relatively a newcomer because it was first discovered only in the 1980s, the diagnostic tests available at majority of hospitals in the beginning was the ELISA which was prone to inaccuracies. Western Blot method or the PCR assays are the confirmatory test for HIV but were not readily available except in some centres.

It was therefore common to sec many patients misdiagnosed as afflicted with AIDS virus while they were not. These days the effect of media reach is so quick, and deep, that AIDS became well known even amongst people living in villages far away from cities. So, people knew about AIDS and that it is sexually transmitted and that there was no cure. When someone was 'misdiagnosed' with AIDS it had devastating consequences on the helpless person because they were outcast from the community much like lepers were outcast in ancient times.

Diagnostic tests produce results. Sometimes they are numbers and sometimes they are images. Doctors are taught to interpret them correctly. Normal persons are expected to have values within a range to be considered normal. But, setting a normal range itself is fraught with danger because these normal ranges are fulfilled only in 95% of the population. 95% of people will have their values within plus or minus 2 standard deviations of the mean value for the population.

This is how the normal ranges are set.

The remaining 5% will be outside the normal range quoted. In other words, 5% of the people who have diagnostic tests will be considered 'abnormal' if you go purely by the lab test numbers.

The trouble with normal ranges is that there is a lot of variation between ethnic populations, geographical locations, age, gender etc. so setting a 'single size fits all' approach fails. You must define normal ranges for each of these sub-groups of the population which takes a lot of time to do. Often, this sort of data accumulates over time and for newly introduced tests they will be found to be lacking and make interpretation more difficult. Diagnostic labs are usually very busy and find such tasks as setting a local population-specific normal range practically impossible except for some of the most pressing parameters.

Normal range data and the problem of 'mislabelling' as 'normal' and abnormal' is more vexing in the case of some diagnostic tests like tumour markers for example. Tumour markers are some biochemical molecules that are present in the blood of patients with cancer. There are many of them available for use in cancer diagnosis, but the problem is that almost all of them are increased in conditions other than cancer also. That means the elevation in the tumour marker levels in the blood is not specific to cancer only. Even non-cancerous conditions also can cause these elevations and it can mislead the doctor if he does not take this into consideration.

About a decade ago there was this story of a guy in the UK who had a test done for diagnosing liver cancer. It was a simple blood test for one of the tumour markers for liver cancer. It was not a biopsy test which would have been far more confirmatory. The test done was a simple biochemical test which is known to be associated with other non-specific causes. This guy did have an elevated level of this biochemical tumour marker and the doctors in the British National Health Service gave him a diagnostic verdict of cancer combining the weight of evidence of his clinical symptoms and the biochemical test report. The patient was devastated. He came to terms with the reality and decided to prepare for the end. He sold his assets and perhaps started writing his will or whatever. He is presumed to have left his job as well.

Then the story took a turn. Though he was doomed to be dying this seemed to be not happening. He decided to call his doctor to enquire why he is still not dying. The doctor repeated the biochemical tumour marker test. The results came back completely unexpected. The level of the liver tumour marker had dramatically dropped in his blood!! It later transpired that he perhaps had an elevation in this tumour marker due to a non-specific, non-tumour cause. This patient had every reason to feel ultra-joyous that he is not going to be dead yet. But strangely, he decided to sue the hospital. Is it for not being dead? The basis of his lawsuit was that he had suffered damages due to the 'wrong' diagnosis not bodily but financially! Poor doctors!!

That is why cancer markers are never to be used for primary diagnosis for presence or absence of cancers in the general population. They are to be used only for high-risk populations who have some symptoms that suggest presence of cancer. In the case of the above patient, he did in fact have some signs and symptoms suggestive of liver cancer. Even better is the application of these tumour markers for monitoring the response to treatment of cancer patients.

It is expected that, with treatment, the levels of the tumour markers in blood will fall and hence may provide a good indication of the response to treatment. In some cases, the tumour markers may fall to normal levels with successful treatment and continued monitoring will help to pick up a rising level suggestive of recurrence of tumour.

The take-home message is that diagnostic tests can be non-specific in that there will always be conditions other than the disease of interest where some sort of alterations can be seen even in absence of the disease in question. This non-specificity is the root cause of the false positive rate of a diagnostic test. If you look at the reliability of some of the crime lab tests like fingerprinting, DNA tests, surveillance camera footage and tests for blood stains etc. there is bound to be a tiny degree of uncertainty in the conclusions drawn.

Even so-called expert witnesses can sometimes present varying conclusions based on the same set of crime lab or other results.

The problem with diagnostic tests is that there is also the variability in results with time of assessments (morning or evening), feeding status, physical activity, method of blood collection, method used for analysis (which varies with analytical machines) etc. This again introduces some uncertainties in the reliability and reproducibility of diagnostic test results. A lay patient can often be seen to be entering into arguments with a lab about how variable the results are from his previous result and what another lab elsewhere gave him.

They are quick to blame the lab for making mistakes because the results are not reproducible. As a lab professional, I deal with such patients too often for my comfort. It is so difficult to make them understand. The worst thing is that they automatically assume that the results produced by the private laboratories are likely to be wrong as opposed to the results from reputed academic hospitals.

The over-reliance of diagnostic tests for diagnosis is said to have taken the charm away from medicine. Medicine was considered an art. The practitioners of medicine used their skills, judgement and experience to get clues about the patient's condition. I suppose this is like the difference between Sherlock Holmes kind of style and the modern detectives. As medical students we were told that some medical conditions can be diagnosed by good doctors even as the patients walk into the clinic!

Observation is the key here.

You must act like a detective who can get a lot of valuable information at the scene of the crime simply by careful observation. A simple physical examination of the body by the doctor can give a lot of diagnostic clues. Whether the patient is jaundiced, oedematous or anaemic, has any rashes or bleeding etc. are vital diagnostic evidence that can nail the culprit. Doctors used to rely on the exact description of the presenting complaint to derive the vital clues. Now the doctors have become so busy or over-reliant on the diagnostic tools that they have stopped being listeners. This is one of the major grievances for the modern patient.

I earlier compared human diseases to social maladies because just like the human society the human body is made up of billions of cells of different types. I argued that problems in cellular cooperation within the body can lead to diseases. What would an economist do to 'diagnose' a social problem? Or what would a politician do to identify the root cause of the social ills?

I do agree that social problems are never for a single individual to solve. There is always a team of experts who sit and discuss the problem. Obviously, they need to know why the problem happened and how they can arrive at the root cause of the problem and what are the 'signs and symptoms' of the society that point to the possible culprits. In many cases the cause of the problem is obvious just as a patient's symptom or sign gives away the diagnosis to the doctor. In some cases, it is not easy like an open and shut case. You need to really do a work-up to finally nail the diagnosis. Poverty, illiteracy, wealth inequality and overpopulation are some of those social diseases for which our societies have been struggling to find the cause!

The surprising thing is that the diagnostic and treatment principles for human diseases are quite like the solutions for social ills. This is an intriguing statement. This fact seems to tell something.

In the next chapter I will delve into the treatment approaches taken by doctors to treat the diseases. Surprisingly, there is a great deal of similarities in the principles behind medical treatments and social problem-solving.

That is intriguing to say the least and vindicates my argument that diseases are 'social' problems of the cellular society.

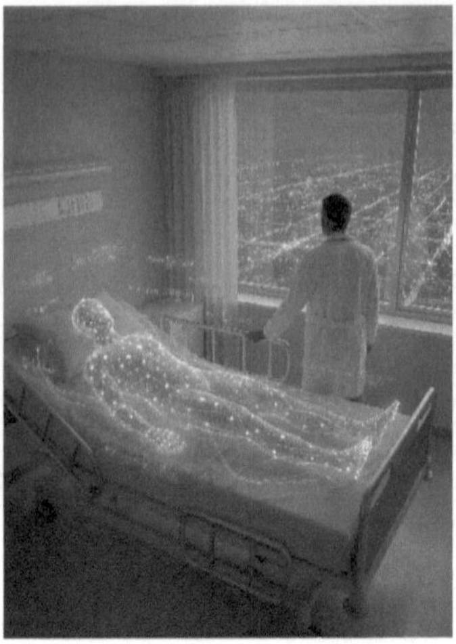

8. Diseases Seen as Problems within the Cellular Societies—How can we Treat Them?

MEDICAL THERAPIES ARE aimed at restoring constancy of the internal environment when the intrinsic compensatory mechanisms have failed. Diseases are treated by doctors in a variety of ways depending on the nature of the disease. There are tens of different medical specialties like Internal Medicine, General Surgery, Paediatrics, Orthopaedics, Anaesthesia, Cardiology etc. and doctors get trained in medical universities to qualify as specialists.

Though there are hundreds of diseases, and tens of medical specialties it is strange that the treatment principles are only a few. This means that you can accommodate all treatment methods into a few types which have a common theme. Invariably, they are all designed to artificially maintaining the homeostasis as much as possible when natural regulatory mechanisms have failed. This might sound difficult to believe.

How is it possible that there are only a few treatment principles in the modern age where medical sciences have advanced so much? This is where this book aims to contribute. I am trying to take a bird's eye view of what is happening. If you cut through the top layers of medical treatment approaches and unravel them in terms of unifying principles suddenly it dawns upon us that modern medicine does not bewilder us anymore. In fact, the treatments for various type of diseases can be grouped under a list that is short—only about 10 to 12.

The surprising this is, as I argued in the previous chapter, that the diagnostic and treatment principles for human diseases are quite like the solutions for social ills. This is an intriguing statement. This means that even social maladies should have a limited number of solutions that could help fix what looks like an infinitude of problems.

An infection that hits the body is no different from a war that the country has waged against an invader. Microbes hit us hard. They are so small that you cannot even see them, but they know how to attack. The stark reminder of this fact is how the Corona virus brought the world at its knees. Apart from the task of mounting an immune war a lot of energy and resources are required for the healing process no different from the rebuilding that is required after a war. An infection can lead to long-lasting harm just as wars do.

A traumatic injury to the human body that requires extensive surgical repair is no different from natural calamities like geological earthquakes (or even bombarding during wars) that need a lot of re-building and restoration!

Nutritional diseases can arise due to lack of food, abnormalities in the gut, parasitic diseases, vitamin deficiencies, mineral deficiencies etc. They are no different from famine that hits nations every now and then and the remedial actions are the same.

'Diagnosing' famine in the society is not difficult, is it? Energy crisis that we see in our society, particularly renewable energy, is synonymous with hunger and related malnutrition.

Social unrest and terrorism are in every sense of the word like the autoimmune diseases we humans suffer from. For a variety of reasons our own blood cells (lymphocytes) attack self-antigens and our own body cells. There are several autoimmune diseases known to man.

Lupus is one such disease.

Rheumatoid arthritis is another autoimmune disease. There are quite a few autoimmune diseases known to us. In general, the underlying principle in origin of autoimmune diseases is that our own lymphocytes start behaving like terrorist attacking and destroying our own body structures no different from the way terrorists go about bombing planes and crowded places. Their justification is their ideology which may be considered misguided.

The fact that this misguided self-attack also prevails in nature in the form of autoimmune diseases is intriguing to say the least. Quite often, the intended target of the lymphocyte is an invading pathogen but strangely the microbe has some 'humanoid' molecule that mimics one of our own molecules. So, the antibody raised against the microbe also damages our own cell that has that molecule. I have elaborated about this later.

Nobel laureate McFarlane Burnet proposed his theory of clonal selection where he postulated that during our earliest stages of our growth all lymphocytes reacting to self-antigens and self-cells are identified and liquidated. This makes sure that our immune warrior cells become tolerant to our own cell types which I guess is no different from the tolerance shown by us all towards our own family members. The problem arises when some lymphocytes become rogue.

Moving on with our comparison of social problems and diseases let me tell you that our nerve diseases are like telecommunication cable defects. In both, the conduction of information is compromised.

When someone has a heart attack there is a power failure in the body as you are unable to circulate oxygen to body cells for combustion. When we run out of glucose or oxygen in our blood our brain can only withstand for about 3 minutes. After that our brain goes out of power irreversibly.

Interestingly, unlike your computers which can be recharged after a period of power shut down, the brain is irreversibly dead after depletion of oxygen energy for as little as 3 minutes. You cannot boot your brain back. Power generation in our society is of paramount importance for the same reason. Our industries and homes will grind to a halt.

Congenital defects are like errors in our project blueprints. They are like batch defects in industrial production lines. You can't do much about but to await 'product recall' from God!

Lung diseases are like crisis in gas supply. Lungs are unable to import oxygen from the environment. The same problem can hit us from related causes like low levels of Haemoglobin and red cells in the blood. Red cells are our 'Oxygen tankers'. Problems with red cells will devastate us no different from what would happen to your industrial economy if your oil tankers got hit. You might think nothing will happen if trucks and tankers go off the road. You are very wrong. You will be surprised how quickly your petrol stations will dry out. You will be stunned to see empty supermarket shelves too soon for your comfort.

There was a time about 20 years ago truck drivers in UK went on a strike. They were protesting and the government did not heed to their demands. Nobody cared to think much about it and all of us went about their daily lives. The truck drivers' strike continued.

Within a week, petrol stations were seeing long queues for petrol. They had to resort to rations and sold only a limited quantity of petrol to each customer! Then a couple of days later you saw 'closed' signs in petrol stations. People could not drive to their work because they had run out of petrol in their cars.

I was very worried how I am going to report to duty as my car had little petrol to last me only for a couple of days. Then I came to know that my boss had not turned up for work because he ran out of petrol. The whole country was on its knees. The government budged to the demands of the truck drivers!

This incident was eye-opening for me. We have come to believe that we live in a society where science and technology has made our lives invincible. This is not true. Our society is as fragile as our body. It takes only three minutes of anoxia (lack of oxygen) for you to kick your bucket irrespective of the fact how rich you are or how much food energy you had in your body.

We are that fragile.

That is why when there is a heart attack or respiratory failure the cellular tankers carrying food and oxygen are stuck in the blood vessels like your vehicles getting stuck on the roads due to roadblocks. It is a roller-coaster ride soon after that and before you know it you are gone. You are on your way to find housing in a cemetery. Your maker awaits you!

I have explained in a later chapter about cancers and how they resemble capitalistic societies. This is all about unequal sharing of resources. Greedy cells take over the entire supply of resources without regard to the needs of normal cells.

This is a typical characteristic of cancer cells.

If you look carefully that is what capitalistic bosses do. They have little time to think about the millions of people who have nothing or, at best, have very little. Doctors treat cancers by surgically excising the cancerous tissue and throwing it out. Or use chemotherapy or radiation to kill the greedy cancer cells. All this vigour in treating greediness is evidently absent when it comes to economy in our society. This is a lesson for us to learn to solve the sociological problem of wealth inequality.

Muscular and bone disorders are like lockdowns. They affect your ability to move in search of food, mate and at the same time evade predators.

Kidney diseases are like making our towns a toxic dumping ground. We need to keep our waste cleared and at the same time make them non-toxic.

Brain diseases are like leadership crisis. Central command is hit. There is no direction coming from the high command and the whole organization collapses. Diagnosing problems in high command is not too difficult both for doctors and the public.

Agreeing that our body ailments mimic our social ills what can we do about them? How do we treat them?

Comparing human diseases to social maladies is where the systemic understanding starts. What would an economist do to 'diagnose' a social problem? Or what would a politician do to identify the root cause of the social ills? Social problems are never for a single individual to solve.

There is always a team of experts who sit and discuss the problem. Obviously, they need to know why the problem happened and how they can arrive at the root cause of the problem and what are the 'signs and symptoms' of the society that point to the possible culprits.

In many cases the causes of the problem are obvious just as a patient's symptom or sign gives away the diagnosis to the doctor. In some cases, it is not easy like an open and shut case. If you were asked what the cause and solution is for a social ill like unemployment leading economists and politicians will offer so many views but there is no single country in the world that does not suffer from this social disease.

This is just one example.

Sociologists and policymakers have the same challenges as the doctor who is grappling with the problem of diagnosing the illness and the ways to treat them.

In order to achieve the above objective of restoring the internal environment of the human body that has been disturbed by a disease process doctors try various means.

The treatment principles adopted are quite predictable and surprisingly reminiscent of the sociological approaches used by policy makers to solve the "social diseases".

i. Maintaining the 'Blood Sea'Transport Routes

This is like maintaining the cargo transport in the world at the right levels. Just imagine what would happen if there was a blockade of all cargo transport in the world, or there was major problem in using the Suez Canal or Panama Canal, or some other major sea cargo route? The economy will take such a hit that within a matter of weeks global economy will be in shambles.

Recently, there was a massive ship that got stuck in the Suez Canal and it caused a 'heart attack' for the globe as this ship blocked the arterial shipping route that was used by hundreds of shipping carriers. The global supply chain was impacted. This is what happens when your blood circulation fails. This can happen if there was a clot blocking the arterial blood supply to the heart engine which disables an efficient circulation of blood. This will slow the circulation so much that adequate delivery of fuel (oxygen) and food nutrients becomes a challenge. Doctors try to treat this condition by clearing the blocks in the heart artery so that the heart engine can pump well. It is basically what a plumber would do if there was a block in your pipes.

Sometimes, the blood circulation is not effective when the person has lost a lot of blood due to some sort of traumatic leak. Doctors would look to replace fluids/blood so that there is enough volume of blood to flow around. You can't use a drying river or canal to ride your boats, can you? Same kind of logistic blockade can happen when an artery inside the brain gets blocked by a blood clot.

We call it a stroke.

Brain is starved of oxygen and food. Brain is much more fragile than other organs. If this blockade is not removed in a matter of minutes irreversible damage starts occurring to the affected parts of the brain. Doctors use thrombolytic drugs (drugs to dissolve blood clots) to clear the arterial block. They act like road transport maintenance service. Same type of clot-busting drugs is used in the treatment of heart attacks too. Despite all the sophisticated modern drugs used for this clot-busting the principle is simple—relieve the block in the arterial tubes. In that sense I suppose the doctor is doing what a plumber did in your house when you had a blocked pipe at your house!

Another analogy is the road maintenance department which hurries to clear traffic jams!

ii. Cellular Famine Relief

When there is an energy crisis, we would focus on supply chains that will ensure availability the fuels and food. Diseases of the gastrointestinal tract often result in to inadequate availability of food supply and doctors do what grocers and supermarket chains do. They source the essential commodities from various suppliers and provide us the nutrients like glucose, amino acid, fatty acid, vitamins, minerals which helps replenish the depleting stocks of cellular food.

Cells can get famished if the person suffers from starvation due to excessive demand for energy and nutrients as in catabolic states like infections, surgeries and even cancer. Doctors effectively work like the Red Cross and other social service organizations by administering adequate nutrition to the needy cells.

iii. Solving the Fuel Crisis

When a patient has a disease of the lungs there is a problem in 'importing' oxygen from the environment.

The same effect could happen if the patient had a heart attack wherein the blood circulation is ineffective in delivering adequate amounts of oxygen fuel to cells far and wide. Or the patient could be having low haemoglobin levels (anaemia) or low number of red cells (oxygen tankers of the body) in which case the outcome will be the same as what would happen if our oil tankers were hit. Provision of oxygen to combust the food is of paramount importance and that is what doctors do. They connect oxygen tubes to the patient or use ventilators to assist in breathing.

When the Corona epidemic struck the world one of the biggest concerns was how hospitals will manage to find enough ventilators to cater to all the infected population. There was also a fear for shortage of oxygen cylinders. Critically ill patients admitted to hospitals will invariably get connected to oxygen supply because shortage of oxygen inside cells will have a profound impact on the vital biological processes.

A while ago I used the analogy of household shopping and grocery supplies. I said you could manage your daily life easily if some non-essential grocery item runs out. For example, no one is going to die if they run out of coffee powder or tea bags or alcoholic beverages. But it is going to be a problem if you ran out of bread or water or vegetables/meat.

Equally bad will be a situation when you ran out of power at your home. Worst of them all is when you run out the 'fuel' of modern life—money. ATP is the energy currency inside the life systems equivalent of your money. Life systems run out of ATP when they run out of food and fuel. Life systems make their own energy inside their cells, and they cannot generate the energy without food and oxygen. So, doctors aim to supply enough oxygen as well as nutrients (in the form of intravenous drips).

Doctors play the role of grocers here. They also play the role of the Energy supplier. I suppose energy crisis is not unknown in our societies. After the Russia-Ukraine war there was shortage of energy supplies to Europe as Russia was a major supplier of gas to Europe. European countries panicked. They had to find other sources for the gas. The cost of energy increased much to the dissatisfaction of the public. A critically ill patient is in the same situation as countries that have their energy and gas supplies compromised.

The solution is the same—find the gas and energy and ensure prompt distribution to the needy cells.

iv. Replenishing 'Cellular Supermarkets'

There are countless number of cellular constituents in our body that fluctuate between tightly controlled ranges. This could be salt levels, glucose levels, minerals, gases etc. When they deviate from the normal range remedial actions are kick-started to restore the normalcy. This includes some physical parameters like body temperature, blood pressure and muscle tone.

Restoration of normalcy by means of coordinated, purpose-oriented cellular processes is collectively called Homeostasis. Doctors pitch in when internal restorative mechanisms fail or are inadequate. They replace, replenish or substitute depleted elements. If someone lost a lot of salt, then he gets an infusion of saline which is basically salt. If someone had low levels of blood glucose, he gets a sugar drip and so on. Because some elements like Sodium, potassium, Calcium, Phosphorus, Magnesium and gases like Oxygen are so vital for essential life processes such remedial actions by doctors help in restoring life functions.

One could imagine the chaos that would descend on the society if items were in short supply in supermarkets or raw materials for essential industries had dried out. I suppose you could also think of bailing out banks by infusing 'free money' to them is a way of keeping money supply in the society intact. If this does not happen the banks don't have the money to lend and the economic engine grinds to a halt.

Your own body 'bails out' the cellular energy banks by releasing energy stored in the form of body fat. Body fat is the Central Bank of the Life systems. Surplus energy is stored in the body fat. On a rainy day when there isn't enough energy floating around inside the body these fat stores are released which in every sense of the word works like how Federal Reserve Bank in the US bailed out the US banks. Doctors supplement this process by providing the nutrients and energy in the form of intravenous infusions. Doctors put on two hats here—that of a grocer and that of a banker.

v. Sartorial Repair of the Body

Surgical restoration of the anatomical relationships of individual organs to enable function is required when there is a problem like traumatic injury and the doctor must think like a tailor.

Or some parts of the body may be inflamed or overgrown or faulty and they need to be removed. In some cases, there may be some blocks or leakage of blood vessels and the surgical doctor must think and act like a plumber as I said before.

Where some bones are fractured leading to scaffolding problems the doctor must act like a construction worker. Accidental trauma is more like an earthquake that has hit the body and that requires extensive re-building.

vi. Cleaning up Cellular Information Processes like an IT Professional

What would an IT professional do if some computer programs go awry? The doctor must think like an IT professional restoring the information links and solve the problems in the software and the associated applications. Cells run a variety of programs that depend on information coming from DNA and the distal information couriers like hormones, growth factors and neurotransmitters. DNA holds the executable codes for body processes.

To execute these codes, the cells require intermediaries. These intermediaries are like information messengers carrying the information held inside the DNA. Hormones, neurotransmitters, growth factors etc. are these information messengers. They are generated inside the cells under the command of the DNA.

When there a problem in the flow of this information, the body's metabolic programs do not run properly and the doctor must wear an IT hat—administering missing informational molecules like hormones such as insulin for diabetes, Thyroxine for hypothyroidism, cortisol for adrenal deficiency and neurotransmitter administration (e.g., L-3,4-

dihydroxyphenylalanine (L-DOPA), the precursor of dopamine, for Parkinson's disease).

Where there is excessive flow of information like hormonal overproduction states (e.g., Overactive thyroids, adrenals etc.) the doctor will deliver drugs that will control overproductions of the hormones to suppress the excessive, unwanted supply of the information. It is amazing to think that hormones, growth factors and other informational molecules inside our body work exactly like our software in an impersonal way.

If you extract the Insulin hormone from another person and inject it into another person, it will work in the same way. In fact, if you extracted the insulin hormone from a pig and administered it to a human it will work. The job of the insulin hormone, or in other words the program written in the form of insulin hormone, is to keep the blood sugar levels under control. Diabetic patients do not make the right quantities of the insulin hormone. Therefore, the metabolic program of keeping the blood sugar under control goes awry.

That is why the blood sugar levels inside the diabetic patient skyrockets. What does the doctor do? He administers the insulin by injection. Effectively, the doctor has installed the insulin software. One can go on listing many other medical treatments where the doctors act like IT professionals fixing molecular software issues.

Hypothyroidism is relatively common condition in the general public. The treatment for this condition is replacement of the missing or deficient thyroid hormone levels. Thyroid hormone is an iodinated amino acid derivative (specifically an iodinated derivative of tyrosine), distinct from peptide hormones like insulin.. It runs a variety of body maintenance programs. Taking the thyroid hormone in the tablet form helps in restoring this software.

Doctors have not thought about these endocrinological treatments in this manner.

vii. Waging Wars with Microbial Enemies

Eliminating sources of infection with antibiotics that are targeted at critical microbial information is a very common medical practice that doctors do daily. They conduct a thorough check on the body by way of a variety of diagnostic tests to identify the offending microbial culprit.

Even as the doctor does this from the outside, your body internally does a very similar espionage operation using its extensive network of immune system. There are immune cells in the body that detect any type of microbe and mount an offensive. There are a variety of molecular ammunition at the disposal of our immune system, and they are used unsparingly.

In most cases, what help the patient to win the infectious battle are not the drugs the doctor used. It is the internal warfare mounted by our immune system that played the bigger role. Whether it is the drug used by the doctor, or the internal molecular ammunition like antibodies, both attack the microbes at their information systems. Generally, antibiotics work in most cases by interfering with the bacterial process of protein synthesis.

Antibiotics hit the protein synthetic factories called Ribosomes. That is where the bacteria assemble their protein molecules (using the DNA executable codes). When this happens, the bacteria are starved of their molecular software (viz. proteins). Some antibiotics work by interfering with the DNA replication so that the bacteria cannot multiply.

Some antibiotics work by interfering with the construction of the bacterial cell walls. This is like a military strategy. Cell walls are like fortresses. They protect the bacteria. If you can interfere with cell wall synthesis, then you expose the bacteria to medical attack.

In the olden times wars were fought by breaching the forts of the enemies. Unknowingly, doctors work like military strategists. After surviving an infection, in majority of the cases, the rebuilding of the body is taken care of by the body's own regenerative system which does a better job than the doctor.

In our societies, wars have cost us millions of precious lives of soldiers and the cost of rebuilding the devastated cities takes even a bigger toll on the economy. Fortunately, for the life systems rebuilding is done internally but doctors assist the process by providing essential nutrition to the patient during the convalescent phase. Usually, the energy needs of the body almost doubles after a major infection.

The body changes from a catabolic to an anabolic state.

viii. Taming the Ferocious Immune System

In many situations doctors try counter-intuitive strategies like using immunosuppressive drugs when there is excessive inflammation going on inside the body. They use agents like immunosuppressives in a range of diseases that result due to overactive immune system with the objective of reducing or preventing the exchange of information between immune cells.

Excessive immune reactions which cause autoimmune disorders (self-attacking immune system) are like terrorism and social unrest. Usually this happens when the level of tolerance to self-cells is broken due to misguided attacks. The doctors try to cure these types of diseases by reining in the unruly immune horse just like governments thwart terrorists by means of espionage and punitive measures.

To be honest, our immune system is like a ferocious beast. It is like our army—it defends us against external threats all the time. But, for some inexplicable reason, the immune system often overkills. I can go as far as saying that it does not know when to stop. Or what is the right amount of force needed to quell an external threat. You do not use a hammer to squash a mosquito.

The immune system often tends to use brute force even for smaller threats. This is not just necessarily after a microbial attack. Even simple injuries we face from time-to-time lead to the same consequence. That is why we find ourselves with painful swellings at the point of injury. This is due to the immune system reaction. The immune system mobilises an army of immune cells like lymphocytes and neutrophils to the site of injury anticipating microbial infiltration at the site of injury.

To do that they widen the blood capillaries which not only allows movement of immune soldiers but also fluid which leads to the swelling. This builds up pressure causing pain. So, you end up with pain and a swelling. What does the doctor do? Prescribes an anti-inflammatory drug like Ibuprofen. It sounds counter-intuitive. You are trying to counter a natural body reaction.

The reality is that use of anti-inflammatory drugs is so widespread which is a stark realisation that our immune system often overacts. One of the most contentious decisions ever faced by the human society was the lockdown following the Corona epidemic. Did we do the right thing when we locked the globe? Global lockdown that we witnessed was unprecedented in terms of sheer magnitude. We grounded all our flights. We shut down all our public places like restaurants, schools and malls. Even a very gifted Hollywood movie script writer would not have come up with this kind of a story even if he had aimed for a Sci-fi movie.

We witnessed it and will tell our grandchildren about it. I guess we acted like our immune system and resorted to an overkill approach. We threw nuclear bombs when you only needed rifles. Medical fraternity forgot that we have a fully equipped immune system inside every single human being that would have taken care the Corona offender. Simple build up of natural immunity would have been enough.

It is difficult to guess the mortality rate if you had resorted to no lockdown approach. Why do I say that we did the wrong thing then? My argument is based on the fact that majority of the people who died of Corona infections due to what is called a Cytokine storm'. This refers to the excessive production of the Cytokines by our immune system while trying to fight the virus. Cytokines are like molecular ammunition.

All types of infections that we face in our lives, not just Corona virus, lead to an activation of certain types of cytokines in certain quantities. Their job is to shoot down the microbe in a literal sense. Within a reasonable degree these cytokines are beneficial. When overproduced they become like a ferocious beast leading to lots of unwanted consequences. These unwanted consequences cripple the body and eventually lead to death. It is true that only those individuals who had a certain type of genetic make-up ended up in this scenario.

Those who did not mount a cytokine storm escaped and survived. What I am trying to say here is that our society unfortunately mounted an excessive, brute force reminiscent of an immune cytokine storm and led to our own downfall. The economic consequences of the lockdown will be felt for decades across all countries.

Human society is now in a debilitated state. We should have used some sort of an anti-inflammatory restraint curbing our lockdowns, but we failed to do so. Politicians failed to do what the doctors do in presence of an overactive immune defence. Doctors use anti-inflammatory drugs. Politicians should have done the same. They should have found a way of dealing with the Corona epidemic in a toned-down way. Our fearful lockdown approaches should have been tempered with more sensible strategies. One might think of stopping all the testing for COVID across the society. This would have cut off the perennial source of fear feed for the media which blew the COVID mania out of proportion. There was absolutely nothing other than Corona statistics in any TV channel or newspaper and the people including politicians were driven to the point of where they assumed that something serious was happening and some drastic, life-changing actions are needed.

Few thought for a moment that this virus had a mortality rate of only 2 or 3 %. With cutting the fear feed people would have had the chance to go about doing their jobs. The politicians may not have been put under pressure to take drastic actions when there was no fearmongering fuelled by the constant COVID test positive figures and the death rates.

ix. Control of Information Flow in Cellular Metabolic 'Chips'

Cellular metabolic programs are in very sense of the word like computer chips. They are etched in molecular language. The metabolic programs can also be analogized to factory assembly lines where the raw material comes in and the workers use the raw material and tinker it in a series of steps to finally get the finished product.

Cells make a lot of biological goods.

There are production pathways for each one of these vital biological goods that are intricately controlled. There are 'Start' and 'Stop' signals for each. Once the check point is passed for each production then it is a no-return, non-stop ride till the end. But the initiation or termination of the metabolic pathways is dependent on several inputs coming from a few cellular sensors. Cells make these biological goods based on the demand and not for profit (unlike in the modern society).

Cells are far more efficient in controlling supply and demand. Doctors try to suppress overproduction of 'harmful' substances in cellular programs like Cholesterol, hormones. E.g., use of therapeutic agents to precisely target overactive biochemical pathways (e.g., statins to inhibit key cholesterol biosynthetic step in patients with hypercholesterolemia, propylthiouracil to inhibit thyroxine biosynthesis in subjects with hyperthyroidism, use of angiotensin-converting enzyme inhibitors and angiotensin receptor blockers in patients with hypertension to block overproduction of blood pressure-causing hormones like aldosterone).

Where there is less production of a biological product (e.g., deficiency of insulin hormone production in diabetic patients) the doctor attempts to replenish the deficient insulin by way of injections. Insulin, like any other hormone, is a molecular program that runs several essential cellular activities.

Doctors correct the situation by administration of the

missing informational agent. If you had a computer what the computer can do is dependent on the programs it has been loaded with. If you do not have Microsoft Office, you cannot run your Word typing or run the Excel or Power point. A lot of cellular functions depend on a number of molecular programs and applications written in the DNA language. Doctors try to administer medicines that will restore the functions by restoring the molecular circuitry.

One could use another analogy to explain this. What would happen if one of the electrical wirings in your house got faulty? We can also look at the computer chips in your computer. What would happen if the electronic circuits were affected? The same thing applies when the molecular circuitry inside the cells is deranged.

You need to set it right.

You need the doctors to do this job by curbing or activating the molecular assembly lines. When a product is overproduced doctors use medicines that will curtail the production lines for these products. This is one of the treatment themes encountered in modern medical practice. I suppose it is like restoring the market stability in economic terms. You do not want product glut nor product deficiency.

Doctors become marketing professionals here controlling the market dynamics inside the body for various cellular goods.

x. Tackling Greedy Cancer Cells and Promoting Cellular Cooperation in Sharing Resources Equally—Anticapitalistic Strategies

Cancer cells are very clever—they know how to subvert normal, innocent cells. They know how to exploit the innocent cells. They know how to siphon the resources for themselves at the expense of the needy cells. In short, they have all the tell-tale marks of a capitalist who is hell-bent on amassing more and more wealth while the needy are suffering.

I explain about cancer cell behaviour in more detail elsewhere. Suffice to say here that cancer cells are killed by doctors by a variety of mechanism that will aim to throw their information content off-balance. It could be at the level of their DNA information (making them unable to use their DNA for multiplication), or at the level of their overactive cellular mechanisms.

Sociologically, we are still unable to do much about concluding about whether Capitalism is good or bad. But in biological systems this is deemed unacceptable. There is growing evidence that seems to suggest that wealth inequality in the society has grown to unacceptable levels in the last 50 years and there is disproportional sharing of natural resources in the world.

This is akin to cancer cells usurping the 'wealth' of the body at the expense of other cells. Doctors do not permit this. They attempt to annihilate the cancer cells by surgery or medical treatments so that they cannot siphon away the cellular riches.

Almost all types of cancer treatments are aimed at starving the cancer cells of their information utilization. Cancer cells struggle to execute their genetic plans to subvert normal cells. One class of anti-cancer drugs include Platinum-based agents. These drugs, once administered, bind to the DNA of the cancer cells such that the DNA is unable to make copies or allow transcription of the executable codes. The cancer cells die deprived of their own information.

Other anticancer agents target the programs that allow the cancer cells to multiply uncontrollably. This is, I suppose, like population control strategies our society adopts when the population reaches critically high limits. I guess doctors here are trying to enforce cellular population control here. They are helping the cellular societies to achieve sustainable growth while at the same time wielding tough sanctions against the greedy cancer cells. Doctors unwittingly become anti-capitalists here.

It is truly amazing how many times doctors do things that smacks of true sociological interventions. Doctors are indeed sociologists albeit for the society of cells.

xi. Correcting Faulty Gene Blueprints

Correction of faulty genetic information through gene therapy. This is one area where modern medicine has not lived up to the initial hype.

People talk of revolutionary changes in the way we can treat genetic diseases, but progress has been very slow. The principle is simple, though. You deliver a good copy of the gene to anyone who has a fault in it. It is like your editing function where you edit your files which have errors in them.

Gene therapy is an editorial function executed by the doctors to edit the errors in the gene files. How many times the doctors play the role of IT professionals? Time and again the theme of medical treatment seems to revolve around information management.

This again reinforces my view that all human diseases have some sort of information failure as their basis.

xii. Tuning the Rhythm of Life

One thing we aim to do in our society is bring uniformity in the lives of people. We call it culture. Culture is a phenomenon where all people in a society behave like others. People behave in a predictable way taking cues from the fellow humans. That is what makes orderly civilization possible.

The human body houses several biological rhythms that run the show of Life. These rhythms keep the cells tuned to the same frequency. They help in the uniform and synchronized functioning of the cells.

The most obvious rhythm is the circadian rhythm which is the Day/Night rhythm entrained by the sunrise and sunset. There are other rhythms that are intrinsically generated within the body like the regular heart beats and the regular breathing.

The rhythmic beating of the heart is triggered by the regular signal generation in the Sino-Atrial node which is an intrinsically excitable tissue in the heart. It generates excitations 72 times a minute non-stop from the moment you are born to the time you settle in your grave.

Sometimes the rhythmic signals pacing the heart beats go awry. Doctors call these cardiac arrhythmias.

Irregular rhythms mean the heart muscle cells cannot work together and pump together synchronously. Doctors try to relieve the erroneous beats by use of artificial pacemakers which will dictate the rhythms of the heart. In other words, doctors are like maestros conducting a symphony orchestra.

Regularity and synchronicity are important in the heart and lung function largely because they are fully automated. Doctors bring the beats back on track. In the brain overactive signalling or firing of nerve cells causes epilepsy also known as Fits or seizures. Doctors must use medicines to suppress the overactive nerve cells just as they used medicines to suppress the overactive immune cells so once suppressed, nerve cells are back on track firing away in unison with other neighbouring neurons. Central nervous system functions, i.e., thinking and actions, are not feasible when the neurons fire irregularly, absolutely out of sync with their neighbours.

This is like members of a symphony orchestra group paying little attention to the master conductor. Rhythmic, synchronous firing of neurons is facilitated by the doctors using pacemakers or artificial electric currents to cancel out the irregular rhythms and allow proper rhythms to set in. Some patients who have had toxic or traumatic damage to the brain cannot breathe spontaneously because the brain centre controlling the respiration is damaged. This brain centre generates a rhythmic firing at the rate of about 12-15 per minute which stimulates the muscles in the chest so that they breathe in and out.

This is an unconscious action fully under the automatic firing of the brain centre. Patients who are unable to generate this rhythmic breathing will be treated by artificial ventilators.

A unifying theme in setting the cellular rhythms right for

optimum function is the need for coherence in cell stimulation. From a sociological point of view, it is very easy to understand why this is important. In our society nothing meaningful will come out of wayward, unruly, out of sync actions by the general public.

People must work together to a common goal. This applies to all walks of life—personal or professional. Imagine playing even a game without an orderly set of rules. Cells too cannot function if there is no orderly cooperation. In some vital cases like heart beats and respiration the body has evolved automated synchrony generators that directs the coordinated function of the heart and lung cells to make the ultimate Life symphony possible.

I have listed 12 medical treatment strategies which, in my opinion, cover most if not all the types of medical treatments used by doctors across the world.

Whether it is a top US hospital or an unknown small hospital in a developing country the principles of medical treatment must fall within one of these 12 types. I suppose, using the comparison I made between diseases and social maladies, sociologists and policy makers may do well to use this approach for solving global issues. I don't think there has been any other such provocative claims made elsewhere likening human diseases to social ills.

Before concluding this chapter, a question popped up in my mind. If you agree that our diseases are akin to social problems and the argument that the solutions to both should be similar, who do you think is doing a good job? The doctor as the curer of diseases or the sociologists/politicians as the curers of societal problems?

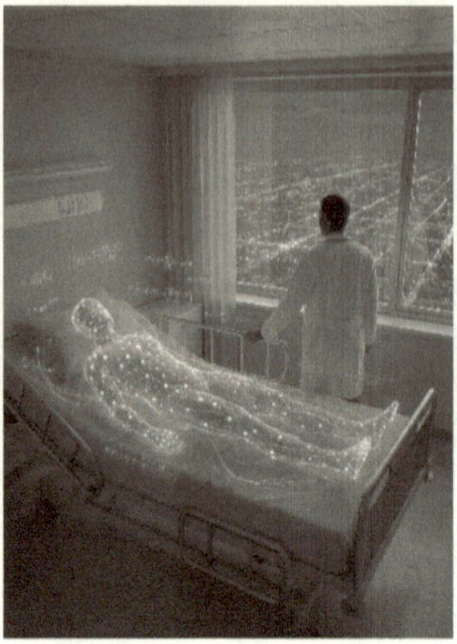

9. Cancer is a Disease that Makes our Cell Primitive and Barbaric

A CANCER IS a perfect example of disordered communication. It manifests unruly behaviour.

Cancer is more about explosion of cellular population. Continuing with the theme of the previous chapter one can view cancer as a social problem of the body where the body faces the consequences of uncontrolled population explosion. Cancer involves uncontrolled multiplication of any type of cell. A cancer cell does not behave like a well-regulated, normal cell. For a start, normal cells are not expected to multiply uncontrollably.

There is a tight control on allowed number of cells in an organ. Our body allows replacement of dead cells or damaged cells to keep the number of cells constant. But the cancer cell knows how to beat these controls. They are devious. The cancer disease leads to the situation that the cellular population is intentionally increased without a due need for it. One can see the problems with population explosion happening in some countries and the globe in general.

Cell numbers in all organs and tissues are tightly controlled by exquisite mechanisms. For example, when you have an injury, there is a localised cellular multiplication to replace the cells that were lost due to the injury. If the injury had caused a discontinuity in your skin, new cells are made just in enough numbers to reseal the skin. All this happens without you wishing it consciously.

There is an incredible amount of fully automated mechanisms involved here with the help of immune cells and fibroblasts. Right from sensing the skin injury, recruitment of cells to the damaged site, turning on gene programs for controlled synthesis of cell repair proteins and growth factors, activation of cell multiplication programs strictly in the region of interest, there is so much happening just less than a millimetre under your skin! Fibroblasts, a type of cells present in a variety of tissues, play a central role in organising these cellular events associated with tissue repair. Fibroblast is, in every sense of the word, a master builder and engineer. It controls so much of tissue building and repair activities at the site of injury for you.

Our bone marrow is a production factory for creating new blood cells daily. Literally billions of blood cells are made every day to replace the dead ones. Truly, the bone marrow can look like an extremely busy factory where new blood cells are 'manufactured' in billions daily. The reason for this enormous 'cell manufacturing' is the short life span of the white blood cells and even the red blood cells. White blood cells (neutrophils) have a circulating lifespan of hours to days. Red blood cells can last for about 120 days. But surprisingly, the host body lives for 70 years! Every single day he or she runs a cell manufacturing plant inside the bone marrow. When this goes out of control you get blood cancer, called Leukaemia. In such a scenario, there is vastly increased production of cells inside the bone marrow that flood the blood stream. At the other extreme, the bone marrow can be diseased due to some sort of fibrotic infiltration, for example, which affects the cell manufacturing ability of the bone marrow. Consequently, the number of cells in circulation reduces which in turn affects the various functions that are carried out by these cells.

Coming back to the topic of controlled cell division, I said the cancer cells lose this ability to shut down the cell division process. Therefore, there is cell multiplication without regard to resources and need. There is an unfair utilisation of nutrients for unnecessary cell division at the cost of normal cells. It is really a case of cellular population expansion with a potential to cause famine for the rest of the cells. That is why cancer patients lose weight, one of the characteristic features that make us clinicians suspect cancer in somebody with no other obvious causes for the patient's complaints.

I suppose cancer depicts a situation like population explosion in a country. There are too many cells to feed. To make matters worse the cells in need of more nutrition are the rapidly multiplying cancer cells. They acquire characteristics that make them smarter than the normal cells. They 'know' how to 'steal' the available cellular riches!

One of the interesting features of a normal cell is its ability to stop multiplying if they reach the boundary of the neighbour cell. This is called the contact inhibition. Tissues or organs can be viewed as a sheet of cells, arranged in a continuous layer. They touch each other on the sides, like our houses are constructed in a row adjoining each other. We cannot squeeze in some new construction between our house and that of your neighbour. You cannot go on building all around the street as you like. If you did that you are behaving exactly as a cancer cell would do. Town planning by the city council is all about orderly construction of buildings in the community. Inside the body there is a lot of cellular and tissue planning as well. Cancer cells do not obey the rules unfortunately.

Cancer cells proliferate uncontrollably because they lose the ability to sense the signals from its external environment, i.e., other fellow cells in your body. Under normal circumstances, a normal cell would respond to molecular signals coming from other cells and behave 'responsibly'.

A cell is surrounded by a cell membrane, which can be viewed as a territorial boundary for it. Its only way of contact with the outside world is through points of contact on this cell membrane. There are specialised molecules called receptors located on the cell membrane whose only job is to sense the external signals coming from cells near and far. In most cases these external signals reach the cells in the form of hormones, growth factors and neurotransmitters. They are the 'information couriers' for the cells who hand-deliver the vital messages coming from the cellular bureaucracy and the body's high command, the brain and the endocrine glands.

In many cells, there are tiny 'gates' on the side of the cell membrane called the gap junctions. Through these gates also they can 'talk' to neighbour cells. I cannot help using this word talk though it sounds very anthropoid. But exchange of signals between cells happens this way without doubt. This information helps the cell to respond to the circumstances prevailing in the body. The *Notch* signalling pathway is uniquely operating in the cell-to-cell physical contact. The peculiarity of the physical cell-to-cell contact as a communication mechanism is that both the message molecules and their receiver molecules are situated on the respective cell surfaces. Unlike the many other different types of molecular messages, the *Notch* systems uses bound messages, which can be decoded by bound receiver molecules on the neighbouring cells. It is believed that the Notch communication system plays a vital role in organ development and differentiation. What differentiation pathway the cells are supposed to take is mediated perhaps by such a direct cell-to-cell communication.

The cancer cells have defective cell-surface receptors. This is usually because of defective signal molecules brought about by mutations in the genes coding for these signal receptor proteins. Information transfer is no longer possible because the system is faulty. Does your radio or T.V work when they develop a malfunction in their aerials?

The outcome of this signal capture failure is disorder in cellular metabolism because the cancer cells do not know when to do what. They do not know when to stop multiplying because their only source of external information is lost. That is why I said in the beginning that cancer represents disordered communication. Just sit back and think for a moment what you would do if you were cut off from your outside world. You are left with no TV, no Radio, no internet etc.

What do you think will happen in our society if people stopped responding to regulatory social laws? What would happen if people behaved as they liked, looting others, invading the lives of other people, keep constructing buildings as they liked and such like? Perhaps it would turn into a primitive, barbaric society.

We should not forget the fact that human beings have lived that way before they reached this point of civilisation. We have learnt to lead orderly lives may be for the past few thousand years only. Still, we do find acts of aggression and unfairness in several situations. But, by and large, they have become more and more uncommon. The world today expects order. If you look at the history of Second World War, it is surprising that Hitler had his way of absolute barbarism for quite a few years before the world could do anything about it. I wonder if the lack of proper communication tools delayed the public outcry against him or that there was corrupt information floating around.

In today's environment it is unlikely any government or political leader in the world can do anything against social order. When ethnic cleansing happened in some countries recently, there was swift mobilisation of public support and other nations intervened immediately. When Pakistan's government was overthrown by the military, there were sanctions against it from US and other countries. When Saddam Hussein invaded Kuwait, he met with instant resistance. I guess intelligence operations as well as common media coverage help us to access information more quickly now than ever before, enabling mass public and governmental pressures. This does not mean wars don't happen. Russia invaded Ukraine for whatever reason in 2022. It made it even worse because it was in the aftermath of the COVID-related economic beleaguering and who wanted another war? But that is exactly what I mean. Disorderliness has no boundaries. Lack of order in this region means that resources will be siphoned to fighting the war, killing people and destroying houses, factories and roads. Unnecessary wastage of resources has the same effect as cancerous stealing of resources which would have been better used by the common man (or cell).

Cancer is a state of cellular disorder, like the kinds of social disorder I mentioned above. It starts locally but spreads quite quickly. Our body has surveillance mechanisms to detect cancer cells as they originate, just as our immune systems fight the microbes. These immune surveillance mechanisms detect cancer cells as 'non-self' and attack them. When the number of cancer cells is low, and especially when some one's immune system is strong, the chances of successfully killing off the cancer cells are much greater. In fact, this may be happening in a lot of people, and they never develop cancer. But even if a few cancer cells escape detection, they can quickly outgrow your capacity to kill them. Some cancer cells do give the slip and beyond a point, anti-cancer strategies are powerless in our body. Then the cancer cells are turned loose as cellular barbarians.

Pathologists are medical specialists who microscopically examine cancer tissues to confirm their cancerous nature. They know how a cancer would look like. A sample of tissue taken from the suspect site is spread out thin on a slide to allow microscopic examination. All human tissues have characteristic appearances under the microscope. A liver cell can be unmistakably identified because pathologists are trained to look for the features associated with a normal liver cell. A bone cell will look different from a liver cell. A muscle cell has its own features and so do all others. When a suspected cancer specimen is examined, the pathologists quickly note that a liver tumour cell does not look like a normal liver cell.

It has tell-tale marks of cancer. They stand out from the normal architecture of normal liver cells. The same applies for all types of tissue cancers. I said a while ago that all types of cells in our body could give rise to cancers. Usually, it is just one type of cell that turns cancerous. It is rare to find more than one type of cancer in a single patient. Perhaps it shows how deadly and selfish cancers are.

Our body cells are quite sophisticated biochemical machines. They have several functions such as the ability to make vital molecules, driven by the information contained in the nucleus. They can make hormones, growth factors, transport proteins, antibody proteins and a host of others. As I said earlier, this capacity to do specialized tasks is acquired during the process of tissue differentiation. This happens during foetal growth itself.

I can only compare this to our professional specialization. We acquire information, knowledge and training to become doctors, engineers, lawyers etc. This happens after a period of common schooling which is common for everyone.

School children are the undifferentiated foetal cells that have the intrinsic ability to become any specialized cell. That is why these undifferentiated foetal cells are called the stem cells. On that basis the school children of every nation are the 'stem cells' that will continuously feed vital workforce to the nation.

The same way embryonic cells acquire specialized capacities by way of selective activation of their gene programs. Depending on the intended cell type desired the cells will be given selective access to a set of gene programs. A kidney cell will get a differential access to some genes, a liver cell will get a different set of gene access and so on. The reason for this 'division of labour' is that no single cell can manage decoding all the 30,000 genes or so that we are endowed with. This is like expecting a school kid to study all subjects instead of specializing in one. How can someone study engineering, medicine, law, information science, business management, and economics together? No human brain can process and digest all the information out there. The same limitation exists for individual human cells. They cannot handle all the 30,000 genes. That is why nature has evolved this system of selective expression of sets of genes in different cells. Collectively, they can accomplish the processing of all the genes. For this each cell type has chosen to process some genes the products of which will be made available for all other cells. The other cells make their individual contributions too.

The cells can make information-rich molecules using their allocated gene programs. These molecules are then dispatched to the locations across the body. Cells can respond to molecular signals from elsewhere, by synthesising and secreting the appropriate receptor molecules. These products, in turn, have biological roles to play and are the products of their own share of allocated gene sets. It is a web, really, of inter-connected functions and it can be broken if some cell failed to do its job. The cancer cells can break this web by failing to do the jobs expected of them.

Before the cells differentiate into specialised types, the cells are unsophisticated. In other words, they are yet to acquire the capacity to make specialised molecules. There is a reason to why cells are unsophisticated in the embryonic stages. All biological information resides in the nucleus. Access to this information is highly regulated. Sometimes, it is not physically possible to access it for certain periods. One such instance is early embryonic development, before organs are formed. During embryonic development, the main priority is in churning out more and more cells so that the foetus can grow and gain more cell numbers quickly. Until the foetus grows to a sufficient size, there is very limited tissue differentiation, if at all. There is a mechanistic reason for it.

In order to have skilled labour you need to a decent number of people first. When your group size was 10 or 15 people in the primitive times then what can you expect your people to be? Can you expect skilled engineers, trained doctors and lawyers while you were living in your cave tens of thousands of years ago? The foetus inside the mother's womb is as primitive as the cavemen. Their job is to first expand the cellular population which needs preferential and exclusive DNA access for making many copies quickly.

Information in the DNA is present in a sequence of nucleotide bases. It is a chain of nucleotide bases, arranged in a unique sequence. DNA has two strands of nucleotides coupled to each other in a complementary manner. Gene transcription is the decoding process by which the information contained in the DNA is used for making products. Replication of DNA is not like this. The purpose of replication is to make identical copies of DNA so that they can be distributed to the daughter cells without bothering about decoding the information. The trouble is the same kind of DNA strand separation is necessary for gene decoding as well as gene copying. That is where the issue of preferential access arises. Which one should get the priority? Is it the gene-copying or gene-decoding function?

This is like files in your computer. You can only do one function at a time with your files. You cannot copy, edit or send the files all at the same time. Only one function can be done at any single point in time. Do you get the point? The same way genes in your cell can be either copied for distributing to daughter cells or transcribed to run the gene programs. You can't do both together at the same time. If the cells try to do both at the same time the responsible gene copy enzyme and gene transcription enzyme will collide with each other on the tracks of DNA like trains travelling on the same track coming from opposite directions.

The cancer cells revert to the unsophisticated state precisely for this reason. Their DNA is occupied by copying enzymes all the time allowing very little access for the decoding enzymes. They cannot make many of the special molecules they could make before they turned cancerous. This means they revert to the embryonic form of existence.

I suppose this is like a society that is too much focussed on useless things like war and terrorism. These destructive activities take over the entire resources and manpower and there is no one to do the work in the factories or fields. Industries suffer and the food production also suffers. There is no one to make the specialised goods that you need. Cancer takes us to that situation. The body is full of cells that have reverted to this primitive existence as if they got transported back in time.

The other problem with reversal to the embryonic, primitive form is their tendency to move away from their location. Embryonic cells have this property normally. It helps them to move spatially and aggregate with other cells to form the organs. This process, called organogenesis, relies on the motile character of embryonic cells. These cells can move because they are not solidly anchored to their base. Anchoring to the base requires the presence of structural molecules on the cell surface to hold the cells pegged to a molecular attachment structure. The embryonic cells lack them with a purpose. Unfortunately, by reverting to the embryonic form, the cancer cells lack them too. The result is liberation of tumour cells into the blood stream. They hitch hike a ride to faraway cellular and organ locations and get settled there. This is the basis of spread of cancer, medically called metastasis. This is the most dangerous part of cancer development. A patient whose cancer has metastasised has little time to live. There is a progressive disorder in organ function to the point of death.

I find this spreading property of cancer a bit like spread of terrorism and misguided principles into the society for their ability to infiltrate the orderly mechanisms of a community. Their disorderly influences are too well known in our society. That is why I said cancer cells are barbarians. They lack sophistication, do not behave in an orderly fashion and fail to communicate properly. When humans behave this way, we call them a primitive society. But, thousands of years of social rules and advances in communication methods have made us learn to bring coherence in our ways of life, which we call as civilisation. If somebody behaved as they like in the modern world, we do not hesitate to call them barbarians. Inside our body, if our cells wanted to call some cell as a barbarian, the choice is simple. It is the cancer cell.

The concept of stem cells is also interesting from the point of view of recurrence of cancer even after treatment. Cancer treatment is expensive and often associated with marked side effects. There are only a few types of cancer that can be treated to satisfactory levels in the sense that patients live longer and are potentially 'cured'. Cancer specialists refer to this as remission of disease because they very well know that the cancer may resurface any day. Even surgical removal of a tumour does not guarantee complete cure, as it is likely that cancer cells may be left in tiny quantities at the site of surgery, which grows back. Or the cancer may have spread to other tissues and organs and removal of the tumour at the primary site does not affect the already spread tumour cells. The reason why cancer recurs is the fact there are a certain number of stem cells that remain within the tumour population that are different from the common progenitor cells that are rapidly dividing away. These cancer stem cells are known to be resistant to conventional chemotherapy and radiotherapy!

We know that even normal body tissues have a supply of stem cells, particularly when the tissue is capable of regeneration. This is prominently seen in the case of blood cells. Blood cells are formed in the bone marrow, and one could readily see stem cells there, along with mature differentiated cells. The cancer also is similar in the sense the cancerous growth is comprised of mature progenitor cells as well as the stem cells. The stem cells are dormant and can spring back to life when the number of mature cells is decreased as after surgical de-bulking or after chemical or radiation treatment. It is almost as if the cancer population is under some sort of dynamic equilibrium.

Another interesting aspect of the cancer cell population is that there is a lot of heterogeneity amongst the cells. The cells are by no means uniform. The billions of cells inside a tumour are diverse. Where does this diversity arise? The answer lies in the fact that cancer cells mutate quite rapidly. There could be as many of hundreds of new mutations inside a cancer cell, even up to 800 or so. These mutations happen in several genes covering a range of cell function from cell signalling, cell adhesion, cytoskeleton etc. These mutations offer small, possibly additive survival advantage to the cancer cell.

A scientific paper published in *Science* journal reported on the genomic landscape of the cancer cells. The team of researchers had looked at 1000s of genes in breast and colon cancer cells with a view to identifying the mutations in them. The team found that, on average, had upwards 80 mutations in a typical cancer cell. These mutations seem to occur more frequently in some genes and less frequently in others. Many of the gene mutations were harmless but some of them promoted cancer initiation and progression. In a way the cancer cells are like microbes, particularly viruses, in that they also behave like single-celled creatures undergoing mutations. This results in changing characteristics in the cancer cell which makes them more potent and less responsive to treatments. COVID 19 virus is a stark reminder the effects of new mutations that made the virus unpredictable in terms of its infectivity and virulence. Cancer cells follow the same approach which makes the work of doctors more difficult.

Very interestingly, the cancer cells can overcome the effects of cancer treatment by way of mutations in the genes targeted by the drugs. Whether you believe it or not cancer cells have evolved a molecular pump called p-glycoprotein that literally pumps out the medically administered cancer drug that entered the cancer cell! The p-glycoprotein acts like a bouncer that kicks out unwanted guests! Can you even believe that? This is one way cancer cells develop resistance to cancer drugs, and it is not the sole mechanism though. Once again, I must point out the fact that even microbes have a similar 'pump' on their cell surface that can eject the antibiotic substances making them immune to the action of the antibiotics? This is one of the mechanisms underlying the antibiotic resistance phenomenon. Surely, it is intriguing to note that cancer cells behave like independent, single-cell creatures while growing inside our body trying to adopt strategies akin to that of microbes ensuring their survival.

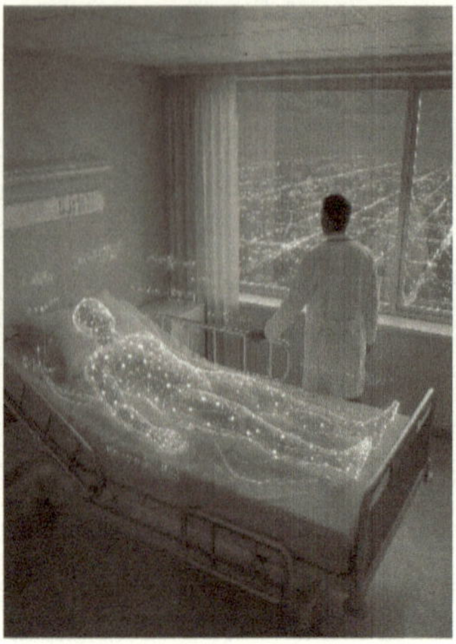

10. Autoimmune Diseases are like Terrorism

WE LIVE IN a world where there are always people who are disgruntled with what is going on the society. There have been many revolutions in history which basically represents some sort of grievance the revolutionaries had against the ruling class or something else. The French Revolution, The Russian Revolution and The Arab Spring are just a few examples of political upheavals spearheaded by revolutionaries who were not happy with the system. Of late we have seen a lot of terrorism based on religious discordance. In fact, the religious intolerance has been the reason for many a war across the history.

Even wars fought for non-religious reasons are to be considered as an offensive by man against man. Rulers invaded lands for the sake of money, gold, women and political ambitions. These wars were attended by destruction on both the sides which to me is terrorism.

Wars, or outright terrorism, come at a social cost. Loss of property, loss of lives and fear take their toll. Today the modern man, despite all material comforts, lives in a state of paranoia. He is constantly afraid some building or plane or bridge will blow up anytime. People living in the US of late have had to grapple with the fear that some random gunman is lurking in their bars, schools or malls waiting to spring upon them.

Why do people damage property? Why do people decide to cause suffering for others? Are we going to live with this self-destructive culture forever? Is it a natural phenomenon? Sadly, it appears to be.

We do not realize that inside your body cells also face this intolerant behaviour from rogue cells. These rogue cells inside our body attack our own innocent cells! How do we know that? We know this because there is a separate class of diseases called 'Autoimmune diseases' in medical lexicon. Millions of people are affected by these types of diseases.

An autoimmune disease results when your own immune cells mistake your own body as foreign. The immune cells, for whatever reason, mistakenly attack the body. The rogue immune cells start attacking cells of our body which were not in their previous 'kill list'. This could be compared to wrong ideologies that terrorists use to justify their behaviour which to them looks perfectly reasonable. The fact that our own immune cells behave like terrorists suggests that after all the so-called 'terrorism' could be a natural, unavoidable phenomenon that you can never hope to get rid of.

Just imagine for a moment a situation that is less serious than religious intolerance or a war. You are living in your hometown. Let us say it is a small town. You would be able to readily identify a newcomer to the town. If you saw someone new walking on your street, you start wondering if he is a visitor with a genuine business or is a crook with unsavoury intentions.

The same way your country is faced with the problem of identifying invaders and culprits all the time. That is why we have the immigration, police force, intelligence wings and even Defence forces. Governments go to extreme steps to catch the unwanted elements. Our own body has the same motif to identify microbes that enter our body, and the immune system kick starts an offensive against the invaders. An army of fighter cells like neutrophils, lymphocytes, macrophages etc. are sent to the scene of the crime. The fact that so many infectious diseases affect man is a testimony to the supremacy of the evasive tactics used by the microbes that fool the immune system. If our immune system was all too powerful, and effective, we would be able to liquidate all microbes before the onset of diseases. But we hardly can say that is true. People with low immunity, like the elderly and those on immunosuppressive medications, are unable to defend themselves against the microbial culprits. Even apparently healthy individuals are seen to be infected with various pathogens at several points in their life. There could be significant morbidity associated with these infections and sometimes mortality too. One could argue that the microbial pathogens are smarter than us because they are able to hit us and cause damage. May be our surveillance mechanisms are insufficient, or our offensive mechanisms are lacking teeth. Or the microbes have gone one step ahead of us and found ways of evading our surveillance and offensive. The latter seems to be the case. Just for the sake of an example the regular Flu virus kills at least half a million people every year!

Normally our immune warriors can identify our own body cells and the invading microbe. In fact, though we are all humans, there is a difference between individuals. It is like the difference in our skin colour, race, religion, language and food. It would be difficult for people to easily mingle with each other and live as a group given all these differences. The same way there are molecular differences on our cell surface depending on our genetic make-up. Though we are all humans another person's immune system could 'view' the cells of another person as 'foreign'. That's why organ transplants are conducted after checking the compatibility of the donor with the recipient by means of the test called HLA typing.

Usually, close relatives may have good match and unrelated people will have a big difference and therefore will not be able to donate organs. If it is done, then the immune system of the recipient will launch against the newly transplanted organ as if it was a foreign invader. The result is organ rejection. That is why doctors take the precaution of administering immunosuppressive drugs beforehand so that the immune system can be put to sleep.

For that matter even the foetus that grows inside the womb is 'foreign' in the eyes of the immune system. But, as can be expected, nature has taken care of this. An extensive amount of immunomodulation happens when the woman is pregnant that helps to avoid an immune attack against the growing foetus. Despite that some women do develop nausea and other intolerance symptoms during pregnancy.

How do we know that our own body is reacting to the 'self'? This can be detected by performing a simple blood test called autoantibodies. This test picks up the level of antibodies in our blood that have the tendency to react to the 'self' and hence the name 'autoimmune antibodies'. Once the initial screening test shows the presence of autoimmune antibodies then the doctor decides to find out the actual cellular targets that are hit. This can be done by further tests that will pinpoint the exact cellular targets. It is surprising to note that all of us will start having autoantibodies in our blood when we start growing old. That shows the ageing immune system is losing its 'eyesight' and perhaps mistakes normal self-cells as foreign.

Rheumatoid arthritis is one such common autoimmune disease condition where the immune system attacks linings of the joints causing painful, swollen joints. Systemic Lupus Erythematosus is another autoimmune disorder where the targets are spread throughout the body like lungs, kidneys, skin, nerves etc. Inflammatory Bowel diseases (such as Crohn's disease and ulcerative colitis) are another common autoimmune disease where the immune system targets the linings of the intestine. Multiple Sclerosis is another condition where the target is the nerve. Even

Diabetes can be caused by self-destructive attack on the insulin-producing cells in the pancreas. Of course, not all forms of diabetes are due to autoimmune causes. Psoriasis is said to be another autoimmune disorder where the immune cells attack the skin. Myasthenia Gravis is a rare autoimmune disease where the target is the muscle. In Grave's disease the target is the Thyroid gland.

The fundamental reason why our immune warriors wrongly hit the self-tissues is strange. In many cases the invading microbes carry on themselves a molecule (called antigen) that mimics a human molecule. I like to call it 'humanoid'. The surface molecules on invaders are like 'face recognition'. When the immune cells 'scan' the offender they look for something equivalent of 'face recognition' or even biometrics. Any molecule that is different from ours, which we expect to be in the case of microbes, the immune cells conclude that it is time to launch an attack. The unsolved mystery is why sometimes the microbes have on their surface a 'humanoid' molecule. When the immune cells see this humanoid molecule and they are not sure if it is 'us' or 'them'. Just to be on the safe side it still launches an attack. The antibody missile made against the microbe (particularly directed against the 'humanoid' molecule) cannot distinguish between the microbial molecule and the one on our own cell. The damage occurs to our own tissues too.

The humanoid molecule on the surface of microbes has been 'stolen' from human cell by those microbes during a previous encounter long time ago. The reason for this is to use the humanoid molecule as a 'forged passport'. Human cells internalize these microbes carrying humanoid molecules thinking that they are really their own molecules.. Two things happen here. One is that the microbe can get into the human cells on some sort of disguise. The second is that an immune attack may be elicited because of the suspicious entrant and any antibodies formed also attack our own molecule because of the similarity between the real molecule and the humanoid molecule. The result is an autoimmune disease.

Streptococcus pyogenes is a bacterium that causes throat

infection in children. What seems like a simple throat infection can progress to serious Rheumatic heart disease in the affected children. S. pyogenes bacteria have a virulence factor called M protein on its surface that is highly antigenic (i.e., capable of eliciting immune attack). It so happens that this M protein is like the heart muscle protein called Myosin. So, antibodies formed by the child against the bacterial M protein also attack the heart muscle because of the similarity. It is like the crossfire in battle where innocent civilians are killed. The end-result is that the child's heart gets damaged leading to rheumatic heart condition. This is a classic example of an autoimmune terror attack.

Generally, the susceptibility to autoimmune diseases is genetically determined. Several gene alterations are identified in people prone to autoimmune attacks. This means that changes in gene programs cause confusion in the immune system in recognition of self from non-self. The 'Clonal Selection Hypothesis' proposed by the Nobel Laureate McFarlane Burnet suggests that our immune system is 'taught' to recognize 'self' during foetal development itself. Any immune cell clone that reacts to 'self' is eliminated.

One of the amazing facts about our immune system is that there is a breed of 'memory cells' that never forgets an enemy invader once encountered. Anytime, even after decades, when the invader reappears the memory cells will come alive again and they will be able to recruit new immune soldiers for the cause of fighting that invader. So, our body has a mechanism by which any such self-reacting immune cells will be silenced forever. The fact that we see so much of autoimmune diseases means that this process of elimination of self-attacking cells is not foolproof. I suppose the clone refers to something equivalent of members of a terrorist outfit. No amount of anti-terrorist initiatives taken by nations can get rid of the problem completely.

Most nations have adopted the approach of using counter-terrorism strategies where the emphasis is on elimination of the terrorists. This is done by a variety of ways ranging from direct drone bombing of terrorist camps, like the US has been doing lately, to subversive tactics like supporting groups that do not get along well with the terrorist outfit that you want to eliminate. In my opinion this is like taking simple pain killers, to relieve a pain which of course helps in the short-term. But a recurrent pain is a sign of something serious and you need to figure out the cause of it rather than seeking temporary relief through pain killers. Governments will do a lot better approaching terrorism as a social malady that needs a permanent cure aimed at the root cause of the problem. They will be better off understanding the basis of the so-called ideology the terrorists are fighting for.

As we move towards densely populated societies people are going to be disgruntled by a lot of things like lack of job opportunities, competition for resources, group identities, wealth inequalities, scarcity of necessities and so on.

Unless we solve that fundamental problem, we will not make the terrorist vanish. Doctors are like the governments in that they are quick to dish out medicines that suppress the immune system to fight the autoimmune diseases. They suppose that by curtailing the immune system they can reduce the harms due to the autoimmune attacks.

It is not that the medics do not know this but the problem in that approach is that the suppressed immune system means your body lies exposed to attacks from other microbial foreign invaders. In fact, some of the commensal microbes (those microbes who normally live in our body without causing any disease) start behaving opportunistically and show their true colours.

Doctors use immunosuppressive steroid drugs to fight autoimmune diseases knowing that it is like a double-edged sword. Are governments right in fighting terrorism with the brute force of the army and police?

Is there another way doctors and governments tackle the self-harm phenomenon? Should we hit the root cause of the problem rather than applying a 'one-size fits all' antagonistic approach to self-offenders? Can we find the root cause (s)? Or this self-directed damage is unavoidable and whatever we do we may find it impossible to prevent it at any cost. This is something that looks like a side-effect of complexity. The human body has evolved to be a whopping 30-trillion cell enterprise.

You don't hope to keep it trouble-free if you had even the faintest idea of how difficult it is to manage a simple organization that has about 100 employees. The same way our societies have now become very complex in terms of not only population size, but the challenges associated with diversity of the resident population as well as the floating population.

We must engage in various forms of international activities including business, border control, war, scientific cooperation, education, and diplomacy. There are numerous cultural identities within and between human societies apart from greedy businessmen and politicians making it a fertile place for disgruntlement.

Autoimmune diseases tell us that terrorism is a natural phenomenon. We may have to learn to live with it making pretentious efforts to solve the problem.

Doctors know that too well.

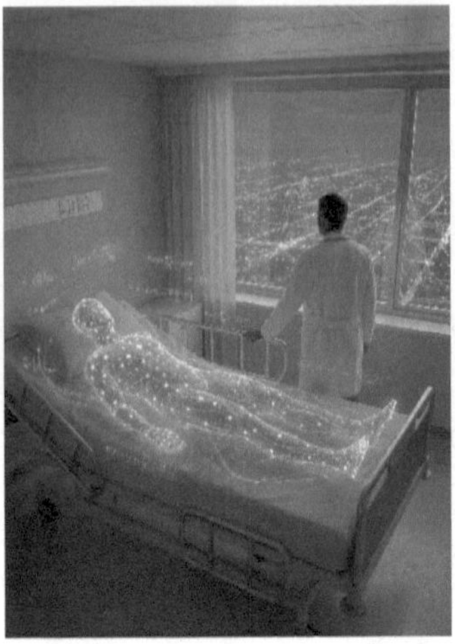

11. Microbial Diseases Represent Biological Warfare

THE WORLD HAS now surrendered to the SARS-Corona virus 19! Also known as COVID-19 the virus has dealt a blow to humanity which will take quite some time for us to recover from. Apart from the toll on human lives, it has probably triggered an economic depression not seen since the turn of the 20th century. Mankind has never seen anything like this in recorded human history. Nobody would have believed it if you had told them that the world will shut down for an indefinite period. It would have taken a very imaginative science fiction writer to have come up with this scenario which we are seeing. We have a great story to tell our grandchildren.

We have seen world wars and countless other wars. People suffered huge consequences during and after the war. But even during the world wars only those countries that were directly involved in the war suffered. Here we are, during peacetime, shutting down air travel completely and we have closed all our malls, restaurants, shops, cinemas and everything all over the world. We have cancelled major sporting events including Olympics, Grand Slam Tennis tournaments etc. We have cancelled the World EXPO event. Just when and why did it all happen?

We pretend to have conquered the world. We pretend to have made huge advances in Medicine, Science and Technology but have taken to our heels hiding inside our homes unable to fight the COVID virus that is so small that you need a microscope to even look at.

This is not the first-time mankind has suffered humiliating damage from invisible enemies. HIV has killed about 35 million people since 1981 and there are another 30 million people still suffering from the disease. Death rates were high in the initial years after the onset of HIV, but as new medicines became available the death rate per year has slowed down. Between 2005 and 2012 the annual global death rate due to HIV has dropped from 2.2 million to 1.6 million which is still a huge number. That is about 4400 people dying of HIV every day!

Spanish Flu (H1N1) virus killed up to 60 million people (higher estimates put it at 100 million) worldwide in 1918 AD. Within 6 months it had killed about 25 million people! COVID 19 has killed less than 0.5 million in the same 6-month period. Spanish Flu had apparently infected about 500 million people which was about a third of the world population living at that time! It infected one in every three humans!

Since the Spanish Flu there have been a few more Flu epidemics. Asian Flu (H2N2 Influenza A) originated also in China and lasted for two years killing up to 2 million people. Almost 70,000 died in the US alone. The Hong Kong Flu (H3N2 of Influenza A virus) hit us in 1968 and killed about 1 - 4 million people worldwide. It killed almost 15% of its resident Hong Kong population (almost 0.5 million) at that time. The Swine Flu (H1N1/09) virus was a recent one that killed up to half a million people in the period 2009 to 2010.

Indian Sanskrit scholars have found records of a disease resembling Flu as far back as 1200 BC! It spread in Southern Asia and Mesopotamia at that time, and no one knows how many people were killed. In 412 BC Greece and Rome suffered from an epidemic that was possibly Flu.

Smallpox virus has killed about 500 million people in a century between 1877 till 1977. This makes it the deadliest killer of man. Back in history, even before this period, we know of the Antonine Plague (180 AD to 190 AD) that hit the Roman Empire and killed up to 10 million people. It is now thought that it was probably Smallpox virus. It came back again around 250—266 AD in Europe to kill a further 1 million. It was called the Plague of Cyprian. Smallpox killed about 2 million Japanese between 735 and 737 AD and it was almost one-third of the total Japanese population at that time! Mexicans suffered in the year 1520 AD when almost 40% of its population died (5-8 million)!

It is just not the viruses alone that cause epidemics. Even bacteria can cause mass human destruction. Cholera bacteria have hit humans repeatedly over the centuries. About 100,000 people were killed in a ten-year period between 1816 and 1826 AD. Similar numbers died in the period between 1829 and 1851 AD. At least 1 million people died of Cholera in Russia and the Ottoman Empire between 1846 and 1860 AD due to Cholera. Almost 600,000 people died of Cholera between 1862 and 1871. 800,000 people died of Cholera again in the period 1899-1923. Cholera is also known as 'Blue death' because the affected patients become bluish due to dehydration and circulatory shock. The cholera bacteria cause life-threatening water loss in the person. They do it by ingenious molecular means that it will leave you stunning. I mentioned this elsewhere and described the molecular details. Suffice to say here that the cholera bacteria keep the 'tap' open in the gut wall by precisely targeting the molecule in the gut wall that controls the water flow out of the gut. The water that was supposed to be reabsorbed from the gut is allowed to escape in the form of fluid stools. Within 12-24 hours of onset of infection the person loses so much fluid that it causes severe dehydration. The volume of blood decreases so much the heart is unable to pump effective volumes of blood leading to shock and death. Cholera bacteria also come in episodic manner and there have been a few outbreaks as mentioned above across the world. Anytime you find recurring outbreaks of infectious diseases you should suspect if the new episode is caused by the same bacteria that has become modified in a way that makes it more virulent. Any immunity that we developed against the bacteria will be useless. Changing nature of the microbes makes it harder for us to develop vaccines as you are trying to fire a moving target.

Another deadly bacterium called Yersinia (that causes Plague) has tortured mankind and possibly influenced human history in a big way by the sheer numbers of people it killed. By far Plague outnumbers the total number of people killed by an infectious disease and the number of times it has come back to haunt us. Yersinia bacteria are probably the deadliest of them all! They are killers. They infect rodents. It then spreads to humans when fleas bite the rodents and then us. The Yersinia bacteria can evade our immune attack by interfering with the function of one of our immune warrior cells called the phagocyte. The phagocyte works by engulfing invading microbe and digests them. This is one of our effective defence mechanisms. Yersinia bacteria know how to beat the phagocyte.

When do you see rodents? They are seen in your homes when you have too much clutter stored in unsanitary conditions. When a whole lot of people live in crowded conditions then these deadly microbes find it easy to infect and spread quickly. When man started living in cities the density of the population increased. Overcrowding was common. The Plague of Justinian swept through Europe and West Asia between 541 and 542 AD and killed 25-100 million people (almost 40-50% of Europe's population at that time). The Black Death killed an estimated 30–60% of Europe's population (estimated 75–200 million deaths globally) in just 7 years between 1346 and 1353 AD. In the years between 1772 AD and 1793 AD a further 2 million succumbed to Plague in Persia. In a ten-year period between 1812 and 1819 AD Plague killed almost 300,000 people in the Ottoman Empire. Plague hit again in a big way in the period 1855—1860 AD killing almost 12 million in India and China alone. To me it looks like nature was finding a way of curtailing the exploding population by means of such deadly diseases.

Typhoid is another infectious disease (caused by the bacterium called Salmonella enterica) that has claimed millions of human lives over the history. It apparently killed 80% of Mexico's population (about 5-15 million) way back in 1545 AD! About 2–3 million people died of Typhus in Russia in the period 1918—1922 AD.

Between 1616 and 1620 AD almost 30-90% of people living in Southern New England died of an infectious illness now thought to be either Yellow Fever, Bubonic Plague, Influenza, Smallpox, Typhus or Hepatitis.

TB is caused by a bacterium. It kills up to 5000 people every day as of now. That would be almost 2 million people dying of TB all around the world every year and this is current data. Malaria kills about 3000 people every day worldwide and this is present day statistics again. TB bacterium called Mycobacteria is another microbe that can work like Yersinia in that even TB bacteria know how to fight the human phagocyte cells. The TB bacteria can reside happily inside the human phagocyte cells! They have evolved mechanisms that will make the phagocytic killing machine sing lullabies for the TB bacteria, and it is up to you whether you want to believe it not. The phagocytes can cause hellish conditions for most other bacteria and other microbes, but they have conceded defeat to the TB microbe. That is why even today TB microbe kills up to 5000 people a day! It is interesting to note that the other deadly bacteria called Yersinia, the one that causes the dreaded plague, also have tackled the phagocytic warfare.

In the past it is said that living conditions in many parts of the world were squalid. This is said to be the case when industrialization started in the 18th century and workers started living in crowded and unsanitary quarters. It made it easy for pathogens to spread easily and unfortunately there were no effective medicines then. That is why there were so many epidemics due to viruses and bacteria in the last two centuries. It does not mean there were no outbreaks before that. The plague hit us in the 5th and 13th century wiping out population by half.

There are so many other epidemics in history which are not mentioned here. The death toll may not be in millions but in thousands or tens of thousands only. I sometimes feel these infectious outbreaks represent simply rivalry between organisms for resources. Or human deaths are the result of unsettled disputes or unresolved 'tolerance' dialogue between organisms. Tiny organisms need the big animals as their home, but our evolved immune system does not allow this easily. There are hundreds of microbes which have learnt to live in unison with their hosts like us. This mutual adaptation is what we call symbiosis or even parasitism. Those microbes that have achieved this have less violent characteristics which means the hosts do not care that much if these microbes wanted to stay in. In some cases, these symbiotic organisms perform some useful function that will benefit the host. Our body is naturally colonized by hundreds of types of microbes on our skin, inside our gut, mouth etc. They are called commensals, or natural flora. They do not cause disease. Strangely, these so-called normal commensals sometimes cause disease in people whose immune system has been compromised. In other words, when someone has very weak immunity due to steroid intake or other reasons these commensals invade the body and cause problems. This suggests that commensal microbes are really playing a see-saw battle with our body keeping the balance and they are opportunistic.

The reason why these viral outbreaks are more common than bacterial outbreaks is probably the fact they are new. By nature, the viruses evolve faster than other forms of life and they keep mutating fast. So, whatever immunity that we develop against them becomes of no use when they come up with new mutations and present new challenges. This is the reason why viral outbreaks come in a series occurring every decade or so.

It is quite possible that long-surviving microbes would have generally found a middle way for hitch-hiking on us without troubling us too much. Majority of these microbes have evolved very sophisticated evasive mechanisms to escape from our immune system. These lowly microbes have got ways of nullifying or inactivating our immune responses by secreting molecules as decoys. It is real.

Interferons are molecular weapons made by us to fight viruses. Viruses can inactivate these interferons by secreting molecules that will bind these interferons as decoys thereby inactivating them. Some organisms alter their external coats so that immune system will be fooled. This is called antigenic variation. So, every time our immune cells organize an attack a microbe their antigenic structure would have changed. This means our immune system will have to start all over again. By that time the emerging microbe would have done the damage.

Some microbes sequester (pull inside) their target surface antigens (microbial molecular structure that attracts the interest of the immune system) when immune attack is imminent. There are microbes that will inhibit the complement system of our immune armoury. Complement system is an elaborate arrangement of several molecules in our immune system that will be working in an orchestrated manner till the microbe is hit. The final effector in this complement cascade will be a set of complement proteins that will insert themselves on the wall of the microbe. I said earlier that this will be like 'stabbing' the microbe to death leading to leakage of internal microbial contents. There are microbes which have evolved mechanisms that will overcome the complement attacks by inhibiting their production or by interfering with their function.

One of the antibiotics called Vancomycin works by a very similar 'stabbing' mechanism. Please note that antibiotics are natural products made by microbes to kill competitors. On that basis Vancomycin, which is made by a soil-living bacterium, is a murder weapon made in nature for genuine killing purposes.

Pathogenic microbes i.e., those microbes that cause disease do so because they have not managed to strike a truce with the host animals. They are too harmful. I never understand the evolutionary logic in virulent microbes. What do they achieve by killing the host or even by causing debilitating disease? Surely, they can never wipe out humanity. Then what is going on? Wouldn't it make more sense if they infected a host and stayed for a long time without killing the host? Evolutionarily speaking infections are like colonisations of foreign lands by people who were looking for a heist. Bacteria do live outside human bodies in a variety of natural settings. Viruses are different in that they are not self-sufficient and cannot survive on their own outside a host for longer than a few days. They need to find a host soon to survive. Bacteria do not have this desperation, and I always wonder why then they infect humans (or even other animals). May be life is cushy inside a host like us as it is a land of plenty. Bacteria find 'milk and honey flowing' all around inside the human body. But why kill a goose that lays the golden egg? Do you see my problem?

I feel the above question needs to be addressed differently. Unicellular life forms like bacteria are the first life forms that originated on earth. They formed at least 1500 million years before the multi-cellular life forms evolved. Ancestors of human species have been around only for the past couple of tens of millions of years. We are in one sense newcomers to the world and may be microbes think this earth is their homeland. We are the new settlers. History is replete with stories of how the native people fought the settlers. I am inclined to view microbial pandemics as one such war waged by them to fight us the new settlers.

Infectious diseases are like wars I said. We fight with several deadly enemies albeit invisible. Before the advent of antibiotics around 1930s and 1940s we were like sitting ducks for the bacteria. We were dying by the scores once some pathogen got into the community. Simple and straightforward infection was proving to be terminal illness for the hapless mankind living all those years until this period when antibiotics were discovered. Now we fear the viruses like the Flu virus and COVID 19 because we have no treatment for them.

Now let us focus on the nature of viruses and the illnesses they cause. What is a viral disease? What are viruses? Viruses are very tiny creatures not even capable of independent existence on their own. They need a host to live inside. They have only a tiny amount of genetic information that can help it to run some programs only. They simply lack all the gene programs that are needed to live a full life on its own like all other decent life forms do. But the gene programs these viruses have are all deadly. They can run a subversive program aimed at hijacking the host cell. That is their primary target. Once into the host cell, and the 'official' take over happens, then the host cell becomes a slave to this invader. The virus sheds its outer protein coat and injects its DNA or RNA into the host cell. Using the host cell's protein synthesis and DNA/RNA machinery the virus makes copies of its own RNA/DNA and proteins and assembles new daughter viruses. These daughter viruses then hatch open and get released into the outside world ready to infect many more hosts. In some cases, the viruses can remain dormant inside the host cells for a long time and in the whole time could be causing more misery to the host. This is more like 'hiding' inside the host which our immune warriors cannot detect. Hepatitis viruses are known to be capable of long dormancy and that is the reason why they can lead to liver cancer eventually in some distant point of time.

The virus that is causing the global scare now, the COVID 19 virus, has got its genetic information held in the form of RNA. As all of us know the RNA is made of 4 types of 'alphabets' (called nucleotide bases). Each nucleotide base is equal to a letter in our language. These nucleotide bases are used in unique sequences to construct genetic information no different from the way we arrange 'letters' to construct meaningful sentences. The COVID 19 virus has 27000 to 32000 nucleotide base 'letters' in its RNA. This is almost like saying the COVID 19 virus has got its gene programs written using 27000—32000 'nucleotide letters'. There are some viruses which are much smaller than that having only a few hundred bases only.

Are 27000 to 32000 RNA letters a decent amount of genetic wealth? How does it compare with other life forms? Are other life forms richer than COVID 19 in terms of its genetic information?

Complexity of life systems is proportional to the amount of genetic information they hold. It is like the material riches we have in our social lives. Some of us are millionaires and some are even billionaires. Whereas some of us do not have even thousands of dollars and some of the most disadvantaged have no more than a few dollars. Lives led by the poor are simple because of this reason. The rich, depending on how rich they are, have a complex lifestyle. Apart from the variety in food they eat they also accumulate a lot of assets and have a whole load of activities needed to maintain those assets. They have their businesses to run and people to manage. Surely, their lives are complex.

How much genetic information is there inside humans? Our human species have 3240 million nucleotide base 'letters'. That is about 100,000 times more genetic information than the COVID 19 virus. Yet, this lowly virus is holding us by the scruff of our neck! How come? Have you ever seen a poor man harassing the rich? You probably can if you know how to hold the rich to ransom. The viruses are simply experts in this game.

Bacteria generally have around 0.5 to 10 million nucleotide base letters in their genome. This is a decent number for a single-celled, free-living organism. For some reason even bacteria have an affinity to 'invade' the human body for whatever survival advantage it may offer. This may be an attempt for a symbiotic or parasitic relation. It can be construed that whether it is the bacteria or virus the sensible relationship should be one where co-habitation of the virus or bacteria inside the human body does not kill the human host. If the host dies, then it would be a loss for the virus/bacteria because they must seek another host. The host would certainly be looking to maul the tiny invaders using their sophisticated immune system. But, in nature, the middle way is always sought. I hit, you hit back, but none of us should kill each other. This is the best set-up. Most symbiotic relations in biology work this way. If this were true, you would not have found pandemics that I had listed before. So many millions would not have died. What is wrong?

Organisms adapt to each other. It takes time and cannot happen overnight. Viruses, like other types of pathogens, can evade the immune attack of the host. This helps them to survive against our immune onslaught. The viruses and bacteria use ingenious methods to achieve this goal. Hosts like us also adapt to the pathogens by developing immunity. It does not look like we have adapted very well yet to viruses like Flu virus because it keeps coming back every couple of decades. The reason behind this could be the fact that the viruses keep mutating at a high rate all the time. This makes it difficult for us to develop proper immunity because the target keeps changing all the time. How can you shoot someone who is moving all the time? The COVID 19 virus is said to have mutated about 200 times within the 6 months of striking the humans. First, it was not a human virus. It was a virus that infects the bats. It may have acquired the ability to infect humans because of some mutation that randomly, unknowingly gave the virus the ability to infect the humans. The pathogens that cause diseases in animals that can be transmitted to humans are known as Zoonosis. COVID-19 virus is one such.

How come viral epidemics, despite killing millions each time, ever come to a halt? Is it because we have successfully treated the viral diseases? Is it because we discovered an effective medicine? Is it because we found a good vaccine? In some cases, like smallpox, measles and polio viruses it is true that effective vaccines were found that helped to fight the viruses. Vaccines for bacterial diseases like TB also helped to some extent though TB continues to kill at the rate of 5000 people a day worldwide. Viral outbreaks come to a halt for two reasons. One, we hosts develop effective immunity. When most of the population develops sufficient immunity, it becomes hard for the virus to spread from one to another. The other reason is that the fast rate of mutations of the viruses may make the virus lose its virulence. It cannot be ruled out though that the new mutations can make the virus more dangerous too. Viral outbreaks tend to occur in spikes with rising and waning numbers of casualties. The changing virulence of the virus may explain this. Each of the peak could be due to renewed vigour from the virus whenever there was a new mutation that enhanced its armamentarium.

There is a school of thought that lockdown during the COVID 19 pandemic was wrong. It limited the number of people infected and did not give opportunity for people to gain immunity. We relied on physical distancing, wearing masks and office closures to contain the virus. While this may have helped to contain the spread of the virus the devastation it has caused to the global economy was too painful. The treatment may prove to be more deadly than the disease itself. It is easy to dismiss loss of human lives as if it meant nothing. But morally it does not feel alright to let people die. Is there any other way out? It does not look so. We could have let the COVID 19 virus run its course till it ran out of steam. It would have run out of steam when lots of people developed immunity. Or it could have happened naturally when the virus mutated out of its virulence. All epidemics we have seen in human history in the last two millennia ended like this. No epidemic ever lasted for ever.

Every couple of decades there are major pandemics hitting us and we have no way of hiding from them. There are several other smaller scale epidemics of viral and bacterial diseases that also keep appearing in various parts of the world like Cholera, Plague, Typhoid, and Malaria. They remain smaller outbreaks because we have some effective medicines for them. But, for viruses, we have no effective cure. We don't even have a cure for the common cold virus which is also a member of the Flu-virus family. Are we going to run each time? Can we learn to live in the middle of these epidemics accepting them as natural events like geological disasters? Can we view them as self-regulatory mechanisms within the earth to control the population? Or can we look at epidemics as warning signs when sanitation or hygiene fell below the mark? Can we see them as price we have to pay for our over-industrialization and globalization which made it easy for the lowly viruses to spread from China to USA or other far corners of the globe in a matter of days?

One thought that comes to my mind is why have we let the viruses gain the upper hand each time? Could we have used our money and knowledge to find ways of beating the viruses rather than spending it fighting meaningless wars?

Could we have used global funds to invent medicines for the deadly diseases like TB, HIV and the likes of COVID 19 instead of allowing the money to accumulate in the coffers of the rich? Just imagine how much progress would have been made in the fight against diseases if governments funded scientists in the universities rather than spending the money on unnecessary politics?

Come to think of it we are spending billions on defence, but our enemies are the other nations. Why do we have to fight the other nations? Can't we live in peace with each other? This is theoretically possible but never happens. Wars keep happening every now and then and cost human lives and money.

These wars are like the epidemics that hit us. Only difference is that the epidemics are cause by different sorts of enemies—the enemies that we cannot even see. So, we have no right to ask or feel sad why epidemics keep happening until we answer the question why wars keep happening where we kill each other of our own type. If you justify wars that kill our own type, then we must accept inter-species war too.

The other thought that comes to my mind is that if we can afford to spend billions to equip us to fight other nations then why wouldn't we spend similar amounts to develop good medicines and vaccines to fight our microbial enemies? I see a big mismatch here between how much we spend to fight humans as opposed to microbes.

People talk of finding a vaccine for COVID 19 as the best thing that happened to humanity. It is thought that it will help solve the whole issue. They say people will at least breathe a sigh of relief and confidently come out of the hiding. But the media is overhyping the importance and even feasibility of a Corona virus vaccine.

A virus that mutates rapidly will always be a challenge for the vaccine researchers. I would even venture as far as going to say that their efforts may prove only partially effective if at all. Even the Flu vaccine that is available today works only one in two people.

At least the new COVID vaccine, when it comes, will go a big way in boosting the psychology of Homo sapiens who have been battered by the media frenzy so much that they have concluded that COVID 19 is the ultimate threat to humanity.

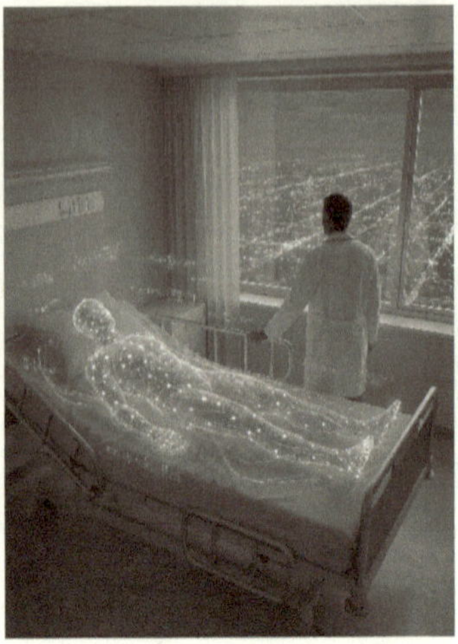

12. Infectious Diseases Occur When Microbes Hack into Our Cellular Information

Let us now look at viral diseases from the information point of view. Flu viruses and all the other viruses are like computer viruses. They use executable codes for striking us at the heart of our cellular information. We all know of so many types of computer viruses that had hit us and all of us therefore use commercially available anti-virus software which is akin to the vaccines that we are desperately seeking for viral outbreaks like COVID 19.

Computer security was lax in the initial decades after the advent of computers. No one took it seriously. But as the computers started to impact on all areas of our life it became glaringly obvious that not much thought has gone into protecting the computers from malwares.

Computer viruses, like real viruses, always must piggyback on something. COVID 19 virus binds to the receptor for ACE2 molecule on lung cells because of its molecular affinity and similarity. All viruses have some human host molecule as the target for piggybacking. The viruses have cleverly evolved molecules like the human molecules for this purpose.

The same way computer viruses are small piece of software that might attach itself to a real computer program that you are using. So, when you open your real computer program the computer virus program also gets activated. It then has the chance to reproduce by attaching to other real computer programs that your computer has.

It is easy for this computer virus to spread like wildfire because almost all of us are using the same operating systems in our computers (what would be called 'Monocultures' in the parlance of microbiology). The *My Doom* computer worm infected approximately 250,000 computers in a single day in 2004!

COVID 19 infected 4 million people as of May 2020 i.e., after 6 months of existence. When the *Melissa* virus struck in 1999 it was so powerful that Microsoft and many companies had to 'lockdown' their email systems through which the virus was piggybacking! In May 2000, the 'I love you' virus had infected about 50 million computers.

The computer viruses communicate between computers using executable codes which are dangerous when a network of computers is involved.

I mentioned earlier that bacteria develop resistance to antibiotics by receiving the 'knowhow' from a competent bacterium through DNA transfer. This is like a software update which we are all used to. For single-celled organisms it is okay to receive or communicate using executable codes such as these. But, for a system that has multiple numbers of cells, particularly in the situation where they are all specialized, such executable code transfer is dangerous.

This is how viruses become dangerous.

In some cases, the virus even makes sure the injected RNA/DNA permanently gets attached to the host genome and this can have unpredictable and dangerous effects on the activation or deactivation of host genes. In some cases, this unwanted insertion of viral DNA into human genome may activate tumours! That is why some viruses cause cancer.

Steve Burbeck, an independent IT consultant, authored a paper called *Complexity and the Evolution of Computing: Biological Principles for Managing Evolving Systems*, which is available at his homepage. The theme of this paper is that the computers collaborate on the Internet much the way cells collaborate in multi-cellular organisms. He argues that computer scientists should learn from the way multi-cellular systems have evolved their communication tools. The basis of his argument is that Internet/Web today involves hundreds of millions of computers in the network and there should be a better way of enabling communications between them. He calls it multi-cellular computing. The challenges of communication and collaboration between networked computers are like those between cells in a multi-cellular organism.

I suspect that this goes for host-pathogen relation as well. How are hosts and pathogens supposed to talk to each other?

About 30 years ago there were only a few computers that communicated directly with others, but now the situation is so different. Burbeck likens evolution of multi-cellular life forms from single cell life forms to evolution of multi-cellular computing from single-cell computing.

I think that is a piece of beautiful thinking. He says that specialisation tends to work against executable code transfer. These days computing machines have become specialised, and you see PCs, PDAs, cell phones (cell phones have computers more powerful than a very high-power computer 15-20 years ago), web cams, bar-code readers, wireless routers, microphones for VOIP telephony, credit card readers etc. on the Net.

Even household appliances have web interfaces so that you can switch on your microwave or coffeemaker 10 minutes before you arrive at your home!

Burbeck claims that the complexity of the machines in the network and the complexity of their interactions provide ever-growing and unanticipated opportunities for hackers. He points out that the testimony to this is the type of IT specialties that have sprung up in the last decade or so. He says that computing epidemiologists seek to identify new viral outbreaks before too much damage occurs. Computing pathologists dissect new computer viruses and worms to see how they work. IT professionals spend a lot of resources on updating viral detection software, modifying firewalls, updating spam filters etc. Burbeck rightly argues that this is so much like the world of multi-cellular life where small viruses and bacteria constantly vie for access to the multi-cellular organisms for exploitation.

The multi cellular organisms, in turn, evolve several immune mechanisms to identify and prevent the microbes from causing damage.

Burbeck's argument is that specialisation of computing machines is also a reason why executable code transfer (like DNA in the case of life systems) is taboo. The fact that each type of computing machine functions in a very different context, using different codes, it simply makes little sense to base multi-cellular computing on transmitting code, says Burbeck.

However, Microsoft's acknowledged ambition to have Windows functionality, Application Program Interfaces (API) and proprietary protocols in every server, PC, cell phone, PDA, MP3 player and game box is the very opposite of specialisation and enables a 'Windows Monoculture' where all machines are similar. A rich ecology of third-party applications relies on the Windows marketplace.

Burbeck feels that this is ripe entry point for worms and infections because, once you infect one machine, spread of the virus is easy. This is like outbreaks of infections (in a community) like Cholera, Plague, AIDS etc. It is so much easy for the microbes to hit all people simultaneously. If many people in the community have the right immunity, they can fight off the infections.

This is called herd immunity.

But, in a community caught off guard, such infections can effectively wipe out majority of the population. History is replete with instances like that. The point to be noted is that these real viral infections only affect a particular type of life system. A virus that affects a chicken or cow or a dog does not have the ability to affect man because the operating system is different. If all life systems had the same operating system, then a single virus can annihilate all of them. Specialization of life systems into multiple species is the ultimate defence against viruses.

Specialization also happens in machines.

Though Bill Gates may want to conquer the entire computing industry with his Microsoft operating system the need for specialization of computer devices drives progress in that direction. Specialisation is yet inevitable despite market forces simply because of technical reasons. Routers (specialised for input/output, query), Web servers (small transactions, throughput), Cluster computers (for parallel operation and more processing power), portable devices like PDAs, cell phones, MP3 players (for low power and long battery life), embedded devices such as in cars (for reliability, durability and precise real time control) etc. are all specialised computing machines.

They all have incompatible requirements and therefore need to be specialised. Secondly, they avoid excess generality thereby reducing the cost and size of software engineering needed for development and maintenance. Most importantly, because the specialised systems support a smaller number of functions it is less exposed to viruses, spy ware etc.

Burbeck says that general-purpose end-user PCs are the ones first infected with such viruses. Specialisation of machines discourages executable code transfer for inter-machine communication because each machine works in a very different context. But a 'Windows monoculture' provides a common context amongst machines with its common APIs. This allows meaningful, but dangerous executable code transfers. But code transfer is losing popularity and a new trend called Service Oriented Architectures (SOA) and Web services is gaining ground.

The point of SOA is that specialisation is possible in multi-cellular computing as specialised computers can rely on other specialised computers for services it does not itself provide. This is identical to the set up inside multi-cellular life forms where all cells need not do everything. Or it is more appropriate to compare them to Bio films, the federal organisation of bacteria living in a community.

To sum up, the take home message is that multi-cellular interacting units in communication with each other must distinguish between executable code and data. Executable code (in the case of life forms it is DNA) is no good to transfer information between cells but perfectly fine for single unit information management. Viruses such as COVID 19 use executable codes and that is why they are dangerous and fast spreading. Our population today is so high, and we all live in densely populated cities, and it makes it so easy for the viruses like COVID 19 to spread so fast.

The Spanish Flu virus apparently infected approximately one third of the world's population in 1918 (0.5 billion): the Earth's total population at that time was only around 1 billion.

These viruses usually are specialized for certain type of host operating systems only.

If it was an animal virus, then the virus will only infect that animal cells. No virus or bacteria can infect all types of animals. For the same reason animal viruses do not infect human cells. Human virus does not hit animal cells. This is because each life system uses a unique operating system in the form of their DNA or RNA. There are some animal viruses that mutate and evolve newer characteristics that will enable them to infect human cells too. COVID 19 was one such virus that was infecting bats and by strange stroke of luck it had mutated to acquire the new-found capacity to infect humans. This happened apparently in a lab in Wuhan where they were studying bat viruses.

Nature protected life systems from getting annihilated by one freak virus or one bacterium all in one go. This was made possible because there are so many types of life forms with highly specialized functions and capabilities. They are like specialized computing machines. Imagine if there was a common operating system that was used by all life forms on the planet then not only humans, but all animals would be infected all at the same time and face annihilation.

Fortunately, nature devised a smart 'anti-microbe' firewall by creating specialized operating systems that cannot be all infected at the same time by one microbe.

If it were not the case not only us but the animals also would be looking to lock down at the same time! Good grief!

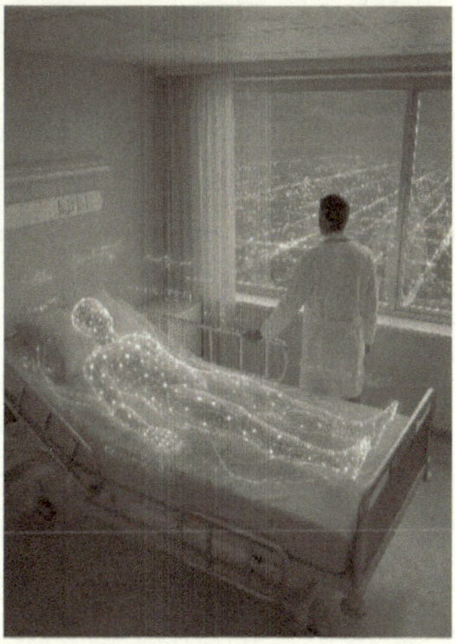

13. Pharmaceutical Companies find Cellular Information Ideal Targets to Hit Diseases

WE DO NOT realise how much of our currently available medical therapy is information-based. The funny thing is that even doctors do not realise this. In fact, none of the medical textbooks implicitly mention this fact.

When you start looking at medical therapy from the perspective of information it is really illuminating and really reinforces my conviction that diseases are the result of failures of cellular information. As a doctor I know that many of the existing therapies can be explained in terms of information.

In addition to my own experience as a practicing doctor I have also seen more evidence for this argument coming from previous job, which was in pharmaceutical research and development. I worked daily with scientists who were involved in the process of discovering new drugs for various diseases. It is incredible that the most predominant focus of their research seems to be cell signalling. It is the hope of the pharmaceutical industry that modulation and or interference of cell signalling are the key to finding better drugs for curing diseases of a diverse nature.

Though I will be using several other examples later in this chapter I feel that a simple example will help to substantiate the concept. Let us look at a diabetic patient. He is being treated with Insulin injection, daily, because his pancreas has failed to produce insulin. By doing this what the doctor is delivering is a piece of biological information that was missing in the patient.

The piece of information that is delivered is the Insulin biochemical code, which is fundamentally important for our body to run critical metabolic programs. Insulin receptors sitting on the surface of the cells transmit the insulin signal to internal cellular effectors once they become occupied with the insulin molecule. I referred to insulin-mediated intracellular signalling pathways, and it is easily one of the most complex in cell biology. Binding of insulin to its receptor activates a cascade of release of second messengers. There are at least 6-9 of them known.

These second messengers carry the information further down into the cell's interior. They alter the functional activity status of at least 50 types of cellular proteins in diverse tissues! Insulin, through its second messenger systems, can affect the activity status of at least 6 different enzymes, 9 genes, and at least 3 carrier proteins.

The biological programs driven by Insulin are not running properly in the insulin-deficient diabetic patient and the doctor does what an information technologist would do. He has rectified the situation by providing the missing Insulin, which is a kind of molecular information. This artificially administered insulin triggers the insulin receptor and activates the cellular programs. Whether it was synthesised insulin or it was derived from animal sources does not matter. All work fine.

Pharmaceutical industries collectively spend in excess of $50 billion a year towards R&D. Individual pharmaceutical companies spend on average 15% of their annual revenues on R&D. A company that earns $30 billion a year will easily spend $3-4 billions on R&D. There is a sustained effort to finding better drugs for treatment of various diseases.

Pharmaceutical companies own patents on some drugs, but the life span of patent rights run out in 20 years. From the time of obtaining the patent the companies spend about 8-12 years, and approximately $1 billion, to collect scientific evidence needed for proving the safety and efficacy of their drug. This evidence is needed for obtaining a license to sell the drug. That leaves hardly 8 years or so for the company to recoup the money spent and make a profit.

When the patent runs out then the drug can be made cheaply by anyone interested as it is not the intellectual property of the parent company anymore. This means that the profits take a steep drop for the company concerned. To prevent the fall in total revenues for the company there is a push to finding newer drugs (with of course new patents) that will bring in fresh revenues. This is the reason for the continuous search for new medical targets within the human body.

Pharmaceutical companies try to identify potential 'hits' that may help them cure diseases. In many cases the new 'target' may offer a better treatment outcome than the conventional targets. In some cases, there may not be any known treatments, and it helps to identify new targets that can meet this need.

Usually, these 'targets' represent the 'Achilles Heel' of the disease process and if we can hit it then you can win the disease. I suppose it is very similar to the way policy makers and economic experts try to solve humanitarian problems. As I said before human diseases are more like our humanitarian social problems.

Poverty, illiteracy, civil wars, terrorism, energy crisis, economic inequalities, sustainable resources, pollution etc. are so much like diseases. You can see hallmarks of these social problems in human diseases. How would governments address these social ills? They will need to know the root causes of the problems and policy makers need to attack these root causes. In that sense pharmaceutical companies do the same thing by looking for the root causes of the diseases.

All big pharmaceutical companies are in this race and quite often the same medical target will be the focus of research at several companies, each spending millions in the hope that their drug will be better even though the difference in safety or efficacy will be marginal in most cases. There is a lot of duplication of effort and resources in pharmaceutical research. This has been a criticism levelled against pharmaceutical companies because this drives up the cost of drug development and obviously the price for the payer.

Drug discovery and development in the pharmaceutical sector is a race, as I said earlier. Whichever company gets the drug out to the market first gets the bigger share of the market. The only exception would be when the first drug into the market had safety problems in which case other drugs of the same class, often coming from other companies, would be selling more.

It is also possible that unsafe drugs would be facing the prospect of withdrawal of their marketing licences, which would be a big blow for the company concerned. Companies are often aware of the competitor drugs for the same disease treatment that are in different stages of discovery and development within other companies. It is not uncommon for companies to start their own research programs in a particular drug class even when they are aware that other companies have already had good head starts.

This often happens even without sufficient evidence that there will be guaranteed improvement in the safety or efficacy profile with the new drugs. These kinds of drugs are referred to as 'me too' drugs because they really are not novel. It has been said that pharmaceutical companies often focus their attention on diseases that are likely to have a big market.

Diseases like diabetes, cancer, arthritis, high cholesterol etc. often chosen by companies because these diseases are seen more in developed countries with the paying potential. There are quite a few diseases for which there are no effective treatments, but the companies often neglect them because the size of the market is small or because these diseases are seen in less developed countries who cannot afford to pay.

Novelty in pharmaceutical research is about identifying new targets. Targets refer to some disease-related molecules in the cell that need to be modified, inhibited or activated to cure the disease. Interestingly, the number of newly identified cellular targets per year has remained constant, between five and six, since the early 1980s. The remaining targets are repeat use of previously known ones. Taking advantage of the progress in genome sequencing and advances in computational methods, as well as techniques like proteomics and genomics, companies are of course making improved attempts at finding new targets.

A survey conducted in 1996 suggested that the total number of molecular targets for drug discovery was in the region of 500. This means that, in the opinion of the drug companies, these were the only molecules that were likely to provide medical benefit when targeted.

A review titled *The Druggable Genome* published in Nature Reviews on Drug Discovery in 2002 suggested that the total estimate of potential targets in the human genome could be between 600- 1500.

We use medicines not only to cure non-infectious diseases but also ones that are caused by microbes. So, naturally, we are interested in finding the targets on microbial genome that can be hit with medicines. If you add these microbial targets as well to the list of targets on human genome one could estimate the total number to around 1700-3000. In other words, potentially, there are up to 3000 molecules in known human and microbial genome that are in some way related to causation of disease and therefore worth pursuing for discovery of new medicines.

If you looked carefully at the types of targets it is very interesting to note that more than 50% of all molecular targets fall under 3 classes—G-protein coupled receptors (GPCR), nuclear receptors, and Ion channels and as you can see these 3 classes of molecules play vital roles in cell signalling. It is no doubt astonishing that half of all new drugs aim to hit cellular information flow. Doesn't that tell us something? This is the reason behind my claim that the pharmaceutical companies strongly believe that cell signalling can be exploited for medical benefits.

Further analysis of the drug targets reveals that over 60% targets are located at the cell surface, which is an indication that they are all involved in some sort of cell-surface signal transduction. It has been claimed that there are probably more than 1000 GPCRs in the human genome. This could mean that pharmaceutical companies are not going to run out of targets soon! Presumably, GPCRs are also occurring in large numbers in other organisms as well. C. elegans, a nematode, has about 19,000 genes of which 5% are GPCRs!

A closer look at the medically interesting targets, from the perspective of the pharmaceutical companies, it becomes even more interesting to note that a large proportion of the remaining 50% targets (those that do not affect the receptors and ion channels directly) also affect cellular information indirectly.

Take the case of drugs that directly attack DNA such as most of the cancer drugs. The main mechanism of action of cytotoxins (drugs that are toxic to cells) is by causing deliberate DNA damage in cancer cells so that the cancer cells will not be able to replicate. It is interesting that these drugs use information destruction principles. The cancer cells were deprived of their genetic information. Note that these drugs do not mediate their effect through any receptors or ion channels. Yet, they hit the source of cellular information at the very fundamental level.

Some of the newer cancer drugs still employ similar DNA damage principles. It could be using analogues of DNA bases like Cytosine that get incorporated in DNA strands during a round of replication. Once incorporated into cancer cell DNA they prevent DNA replication, as these analogues of DNA bases do not allow the copying enzymes to work well. The consequence is that new cancer cells cannot form. Other types of DNA damaging cancer drugs use inhibitors of enzymes like Thymidylate Synthase that is required for synthesis for DNA bases. By doing it we are literally starving the cancer cells of raw materials for making DNA and therefore the cells are starved of the genetic information. Another very commonly used medicine for cancer is platinum. Platinum-based cancer medicines damage DNA by forming covalent crosslinks (adducts) with DNA strands, preventing proper replication of cancer cells. These drugs are powerful and effective.

Looking at the biochemical classes of current pharmacological targets it is also worth mentioning that a very significant number of them are enzymes, mostly proteases (enzymes that cleave proteins), reverse transcriptase (like enzymes in HIV virus that can reverse-copy DNA), kinases (enzymes that can attach a phosphate group to a molecule), DNA polymerase (enzyme that can copy DNA), phosphatases (enzyme that can remove attached phosphate group from a molecule), phosphodiesterase, ribonucleases (enzyme that can breakdown RNA) etc. It is readily apparent that these enzyme classes play vital roles in biochemical signalling. These drugs were not included in the direct receptor or ion channel targets as their mechanism of action is distal (downstream) to the activation of receptors or ion channels.

Here is an example.

The importance of phosphorylation/dephosphorylation in cell signalling is well known and it is no wonder that kinases (phosphorylating enzymes) and phosphatases (dephosphorylation enzymes that enable phosphate removal) score high on the list of medical targets.

In biochemistry of living organisms, attachment of a phosphate group to the surface of a molecule (like a receptor or an enzyme) is a reversible signal to activate or deactivate a particular step. The attached phosphate group can be removed when the said action needs to be reversed.

There are literally tens of instances where cells regulate their internal biochemistry by way of the reversible phosphorylation/dephosphorylation reactions. So much of biochemical meaning is attached to this rather widespread mechanism of cell signalling. It is almost like a 'transistor' in computer chips which determines the 'on/off' status. Phosphorylation could mean 'on' and dephosphorylation means 'off' and what a way to reversibly signal certain reactions inside the cell? These phosphorylation/dephosphorylation enzymes are naturally sought after as potential targets amenable for pharmacological modulation.

Polymerase is the enzyme that copies DNA and Ribonuclease is the enzyme that degrades RNA. Since both play crucial roles in genetic information one can see how drugs targeting these enzymes could modulate/interfere with genetic information. Proteases and reverse transcriptase play a role in HIV replication and are therefore inhibitors of these two enzymes are very useful drugs in HIV treatment. Reverse transcriptase is the enzyme that allows integration of the HIV RNA, after conversion to DNA, into the human DNA.

By preventing this step what we are achieving is an inhibition of viral DNA from copying and multiplying. Basically, HIV viruses are denied the ability to use their own information.

i. Information-Targeted Therapies

Receptors, as I said right from the beginning of this chapter, are the most frequent and obvious targets if you wanted to garble abnormal cell signalling. This is the age of targeted therapies where you hit the diseased cell with a precision-controlled drug. In other words, these modern targeted drugs act like guided missiles. They hit exactly where you want them to hit.

It is not surprising that often we want to hit information transfer mechanisms aimed at the cell-surface receptors. Cancer treatment in the past was very messy. Many of the agents were like crude bombs. You gave these highly toxic drugs to the cancer patients who would unfortunately face side effects that would sometimes drastically lower the quality of the short life that was left. In many cases the dying patient simply wants to be left alone. You would often see people lose hair, have serious falls in blood cell counts, get diarrhoea and malabsorption etc. This was because the old-fashioned cancer drugs attacked not only the cancer cells but also the normal cells, which were caught in crossfire.

Some of the newer cancer agents also work by other interesting ways. They can block information transfer between cells that occur through growth factors and their respective receptors. Growth factors are vital for growth of cells and rapidly dividing cancer cell need more of them. Various growth factors like epidermal growth factor, fibroblast growth factor, vascular endothelial growth factor, platelet-derived growth factor are critical informational molecules in cell growth.

Pharmaceutical companies devised inhibitors of the receptors for these growth factors, and they seem to do very well in treatment of cancer. Several pharmaceutical companies are actively studying several cancer drugs that can inhibit more than one type of growth factor receptors.

For example, some of the novel treatments for cancer target epidermal growth factor as well as other growth factors like vascular endothelial growth factor. The number of receptor types that be targeted can be sometimes as many as four. The thinking behind this strategy is to hit at as many signal transfer points as possible to maximise the effects of information garbling.

Targeted cancer therapies are conceptually similar to the guided ballistic missiles we use on modern warfare today.

ii. Targeting Intracellular Information Couriers

The growth factor receptors mediate their intracellular signalling using mostly tyrosine phosphorylation mechanism and therefore the drugs of this class are tyrosine kinase inhibitors. In simple terms attachment of phosphate group to tyrosine amino acid on a protein

(Tyrosine Kinase) is said to carry a huge biological role and interfering with this phosphate addition step has become a highly rewarding pharmaceutical strategy.

Herceptin (trastuzumab) is a monoclonal antibody targeting the HER2 receptor, used as an example of targeted therapy that inhibits cellular information transfer happening through the Epidermal Growth Factor. Herceptin has transformed the way breast cancer is treated these days.

In addition to DNA damage and inhibition of Tyrosine kinase-based growth factor receptors there are other approaches as well that have been employed to kill the cancer cell. One such mechanism is to inhibit specific intracellular second messengers involved in signal transduction other than these tyrosine kinases. There are a few types of kinase inhibitors currently in use and in development.

Examples include inhibitors of Serine/Threonine Kinases such as Mitogen-activated protein kinase, Jun Kinase and Cyclin-dependent kinase. In many types of cancer these intracellular signalling pathways are deranged. They usually get activated at a rate that is higher than usually seen in the normal cells. Interestingly, in many instances, there is a constitutive (permanent) activation of these pathways due to mutations in the receptors or oversupply of relevant stimulatory growth factors that keep these intracellular signal transduction pathways always active.

The kinds of mutations I mentioned in the previous paragraph seen in cancer cells can be viewed as if some tap is purposely and intentionally kept open always. One can also compare this with purposely keeping an important entry gate always open and unguarded.

Cancer cells are cunning. They know how to manipulate the controls and checkpoints. The word 'know' may sound too anthropological, but when you must describe what we observe in reality one cannot avoid this.

iii. Slowing Down Cell Divisions to Solve Cellular Population Explosions

Cyclin-dependent kinase is a mediator of cell cycle control and is activated by unique cell cycle control proteins called cyclins. A cyclical process, with rigid checkpoints, tightly controls normal cell division.

The basic purpose of a cell cycle is to allow a cell to undergo controlled division to produce an offspring cell. This is needed in practically most types of cells in our body except perhaps in the case of nerve cells. Skin cells may need to multiply and form new cells if there is an injury to skin. Hair cells need to multiply to replace lost hair. Many cell types in our body have a finite life span and the dying ones need to be replaced. There are some cell types in our body that divide more often than others. Cancer is the condition where the cells have lost the regulatory control and so divide uncontrollably without regard to need and availability of resources to support the newly formed cells.

Cell cycle itself is comprised of distinct stages, which must run one after another. The cell cannot move to the next stage before the previous one is completed.

The book *Molecular Biology of the Cell* edited by Alberts et al compares the cell cycle to the control system of automatic washing machine. A clock, or a timer, turns on each event at a specific time allowing a fixed amount of time for each event. The essential processes in the wash cycle occur in stages: it takes in water, mixes it with detergent, washes the clothes, rinses them, and spins them dry.

There is mechanism to initiate events in the correct order and allow them to happen only once per cycle. Sensors detect completion of each step and can delay progression to next step if the previous step is not yet complete due to a malfunction. In our cells the cell cycle is also controlled by such sensors, which put a block on the progression of cell division if a fault is detected. These checkpoints make sure that cell is not undergoing runaway cell divisions.

Cancer cells can overcome these checkpoints by making mutated versions of the checkpoint molecules that are no more susceptible to the regulatory action. Therefore, the cancer cells can undergo uncontrolled cell divisions. As one can imagine inhibitors of the Cyclin-mediated signalling are being currently evaluated for cancer treatment.

iv. Tumour Suppressors

Our body has some interesting molecules whose role is to suppress tumour development. An example is the BRCA1 gene that is known to be associated with breast cancer development. Women who inherit one mutant BRCA1 allele have a 60% probability of developing breast cancer by the age of 50. The other tumour suppressor gene known is the APC gene. Mutant APC gene is known to predispose to colon cancer. What do the tumour suppressor genes do? Their role is to prevent uncontrolled cell divisions. They slow down or inhibit the progression of cell through a specific stage of the cell cycle. Cancer cells seem to subvert these checkpoints such that the cell divisions happen unchecked.

I suppose it is like capitalists who subvert all governmental controls in evading taxation also moral responsibility. Unchecked proliferation of capitalistic businesses affects governmental revenue which, if received properly, would help in welfare projects for the citizens. Instead, the capitalistic bosses evade payment of taxes by moving their registered headquarters to a tax haven country. Apart from evaded tax these companies also escape from other governmental regulations because they argue that they are registered in a different country.

Cancer cells do the same. They 'know' how to deceive the system and go for uncontrolled cell proliferation of these mutated, good for nothing cancer cells, at the expense of other needy cells. Conceptually, I am sure readers would understand how big businesses continue to expand to all geographies (metastasis) and reap the profits which could have gone to small, legitimate businesses in those regions.

A protein called p53 can be termed the ultimate tumour suppressor in our cells. Inactivation of its tumour-suppressor activity is almost a universal step in the development of human cancers.

This is like the multinational corporations subverting the governmental regulations to proliferate all over the world. Because p53 protects the cells from becoming cancerous the p53 protein has also been termed 'the guardian of the genome'. Pharmaceutical companies are trying desperately to exploit p53 as a medical target, but no company has succeeded yet.

In some cancers it is well known that the tumour cells need the action of hormones to enable the growth and division of the cells.

For example, the breast cancer cells need oestrogen hormone to survive and grow. This is the basis for using Oestrogen antagonists for treatment of breast cancer. A classic example would be Tamoxifen, which revolutionised the treatment of breast cancer. Prostate cancer requires male sex hormone (Testosterone) for its growth and that is why Testosterone antagonists are useful for treatment of prostate cancer. This is curiously different from providing hormones for treatment of some diseases like diabetes. Either way, the result that is achieved touches upon the theme of biochemical signalling. It must be pointed out here that women are treated with oestrogen supplements as part of the hormone replacement therapy because, with old age, the ovaries lose the ability to generate oestrogen. This context is akin to replacement of Insulin in diabetics.

The problem with HRT is that oestrogen can produce some unwanted effects that have been highly debated over the years like the risk of breast cancer etc.

v. One Signal, Many Decoders and Multiple Pharmacological Options

Receptor inhibition, and the consequent arrest of intracellular signal transfer, is not limited to treatment of cancer. Pharmaceutical companies have adopted this approach for treatment of several disease types.

The drugs you take for even common conditions like Hay fever and other allergies are interceptors of biological information. Antihistamines block the action of Histamine that gets released by mast cells (cells that play important roles in allergy). Histamine produces dilation of blood vessels and several other actions that promote allergy by acting through type 1 histamine receptor. Specifically, these histamine-blocking drugs block the histamine-mediated signalling through this type 1 receptor.

Interestingly, histamine also plays a role in acid secretion in your stomach assisting the digestive process. This effect is mediated by type 2 histamine receptors. Blockers of type 2 histamine receptors are big-time sellers belonging to the class of drugs called antacids. They are very useful for the treatment of peptic ulcer.

Honestly, I do not think most readers would have associated simple allergy medication and antacid medication with information blockade. But the truth is that is what they are. The purpose of this chapter is to show that many, if not most, of the drugs are blockers of information flow.

You need to think of receptors as molecular receivers. For your phone and TV communication you may use satellite dishes and aerials. Cells do not have those technologies. Instead, they rely on receptors stationed on cell surface. These receptors are designed specific to recognize and bind messenger molecules. Generally, one receptor type for one messenger type exists. This brings about specificity in cell-cell communication. The receptors and the corresponding messenger molecules fit like a lock and key. Once this binding happens the receptor molecule undergoes further steps in activation which may involve structural changes on receptor structure or activation of a second messenger inside the cell which will carry the signal inside.

Receptor multiplicity is a common biological phenomenon. This is a way of accomplishing multiple cell responses with a single type of signal. From the medical perspective it becomes necessary to target individual receptor subtypes when you want to affect one of these multiple cell responses. I suppose the more important examples of receptor multiplicity, from medical point of view, are dopamine, adrenaline, serotonin (5-hydroxytryptamine) etc. 5-hydroxytryptamine (5-HT) receptors come in at least 14 forms, the highest for any informational molecule! Dopamine receptors occur in 5 types!

The advantage of multiple receptor types is that each of these receptor types is situated on different organs and tissues. Each organ or tissue will have only one type of the receptor. I said above that serotonin receptors exist in 14 forms! That means there are 14 cell types in our body which can recognize and decode the serotonin signal.

The interesting thing is that each of these 14 cells that respond to serotonin signals would produce slightly different effects because of their receptor variation. This is a biological curiosity. Nature has achieved what our modern communication technology cannot do. By enabling differential cell responses in 14 different cell types, serotonin signal can produce multiple effects which, very interestingly, will complement each other towards a common goal.

Let me explain this intriguing concept a bit more using another example.

Adrenaline receptors are basically of two types—alpha and beta. Alpha and beta adrenaline receptors can occur in more than one form again - alpha 1 and 2, beta 1 and 2 etc. I will now restrict my discussion to medical applications of these receptor subtypes. Alpha adrenaline receptors mediate constriction of blood vessels. In medical situations where the blood pressure is low, due to blood loss etc. it is helpful to purposely narrow the blood vessel lumen with drugs that can stimulate vasoconstriction. Vasoconstriction raises the blood pressure and enables better circulation of blood.

If someone loses a lot of blood the blood vessels do not fill up fully. The heart is unable to keep enough blood in circulation and the blood pressure falls low. What the doctors do, apart from infusion of blood or saline to expand the blood volume, is to use drugs like noradrenaline, which is an alpha 1 adrenaline receptor activator. This will lead to constriction of the blood vessels and an increase in blood pressure.

Such drugs are also used in situations like septic shock when the blood pressure falls low due to blood vessels dilating. This is due to release of several molecules involved in the immune process. In this disease setting, potentially life threatening, the problem is not loss of blood but a fall in blood pressure due to dilated blood vessels.

As one can imagine, alpha adrenaline receptors become the target if you want to lower the blood pressure as well. But, in this instance, the drugs to lower blood pressure will be inhibitors of the alpha-receptor and not activators. By inhibiting the receptor, the vessels are prevented from constricting. Instead, they become dilated thereby reducing the pressure inside the blood vessels.

Beta 2 adrenaline receptor mediates the effect of dilation of the bronchi in your lungs in response to signals coming in the form of adrenaline. This allows us to breathe heavily to meet emergencies. This pharmacological effect is exploited by use of stimulators of beta 2 adrenaline receptor like salbutamol for treatment of asthma.

Blockers of beta 1 adrenaline receptors come handy when you want to reduce the heart rate to lower the effort the heart needs to make towards contraction. Heart muscle contraction is an energy requiring activity and requires a lot of blood flow through the heart muscle. In situations like heart attack the heart muscle undergoes ischemic damage and struggles to beat with sufficient force. Beta adrenaline receptor blockers come handy by enabling a lowering of the rate of the heart beats and therefore save the heart muscle from over activity. That is why drugs like beta-blockers are widely used for treatment of patients who have suffered a heart attack. They are also used for treatment of people with high blood pressure for the same reason.

In fact, they are also used to treat symptoms of anxiety. Anxiety leads to rapid fluttering of the heart and beta-blockers are useful to control this. It is also known that some people use beta-blockers to control symptoms of stage fright. When they must make a public speech they take beta- blockers beforehand to help them to control their rapid heartbeats!

As one can see adrenaline signal helps to activate multiple types of cell responses that all add up towards a common goal. Imagine you are in a danger.

Let us say you are being attacked by a animal or a stranger.

You need to be able to pump blood in your heart fast enough which is taken care of by the specific type of adrenaline receptor in heart muscle. You need to make sure you lose less blood in a bloody conflict. Adrenaline receptor subtype present on vessel walls will ensure constriction of the blood vessels so that you do not bleed a lot. You are going to need a lot of oxygen to supply fuel to the rest of the body including your muscles which need to contract rapidly to help in running or fighting. Adrenaline receptor subtype in your bronchi will help in dilating the bronchi.

From a functional point of view, I suppose readers now understand how nature uses minimalistic designs to achieve great results. In medical science doctors now use drugs that preferentially activate or block specific receptor subtypes which means you can target a specific biological function.

As I said above adrenaline receptor blockers and activators have a role in treating hypotension, tachycardia/bradycardia (increase or decrease in heart rate), asthma etc.

The common theme is cell signalling and medical ways of interfering with this signalling.

In the case of 5 HT receptors, it is curious to note that each type of receptors mediates different effect. Pharmaceutical companies who have discovered specific blockers or activators of sub types of 5HT receptors exploit this. Antipsychotic drugs like Clozapine, used in treatment of Schizophrenia, are a more selective antagonist of 5-HT_{2A}, 5-HT2C and 5-HT_6 receptors. Interestingly, these types of newer antipsychotic agents also target dopamine receptors (especially D2 and D4 types). As you can see the drugs have a broad specificity towards different signalling systems in the brain by affecting more than one neurotransmitter signal.

Even more interestingly, 5-HT_3 receptors mediate completely different biological process, namely mediation of vomiting response. Antagonists of this 5-HT receptor subtype have been developed by pharmaceutical companies to control severe vomiting seen in seriously ill patients. Particularly cancer patients on treatment with highly toxic cancer drugs have serious vomiting and 5-HT blockers are useful in this setting.

Triptans are selective 5-HT1B/1D receptor agonists are powerful medicines for treatment of a completely different disease—migraine! Stimulation of 5-HT_4 with drugs like Mosapride helps in the treatment of constipation-predominant irritable bowel syndrome! One signal, many receptors, many diseases and multiple drugs!

vi. Drugs that will Support Homeostatic Balance

A fall in salt concentration in the blood will cause a fall in the extra cellular volume, which includes the intra vascular blood volume, which will affect the circulatory system in terms of efficient transport of nutrients and oxygen. To prevent this from happening adaptive responses kick in with an overall objective of bringing the vascular and extra cellular volume back to the original level.

Afferent signals (incoming) captured by arterial baroreceptor cells (sensors on the wall of the arteries that will capture the blood pressure), atrial stretch receptors (sensors on the wall of the heart chambers that will sense the internal pressure by means of the amount of stretch), intra-renal baroreceptor cells (sensors located at a different place in this case inside the kidneys that will capture the blood pressure) and intra-thoracic volume receptors trigger the release of renin by the juxtaglomerular cells of the nephrons.

Renin is an enzyme that can act on hormonally inactive angiotensinogen released by the liver to produce angiotensin I, which is a 10-amino acid long protein. Further steps are required to generate information out of this molecule which involves removal of two amino acids from one end, cleaved by the angiotensin-converting enzyme, produced by a variety of cells such as vascular endothelium, lung, liver, adrenal cortex, kidney, and neurohypophysis to synthesise angiotensin II which is information-rich.

Angiotensin II can bind specific receptors on target cells and stimulate the rate-limiting steps of aldosterone synthesis by the adrenal cortical cells to release aldosterone, which is another information-rich molecule. Aldosterone (a hormone) will carry a message to the renal distal tubular cells, decoded by the aldosterone receptors on these target cells, to conserve salt.

Angiotensin II also has other secondary actions on other cells like myocardium (enhanced myocardial contraction), vascular smooth muscle cells (vasoconstriction), intestinal cells (salt and water reabsorption) and neural centres in hypothalamus (thirst and salt appetite) and, as one can see, these actions lead to a common goal of expansion of blood volume and an efficient circulation.

I suppose Renin-Angiotensin axis in our body is another good example of one signal—multiple coordinated effects. In this case the fall in salt levels in the body, and the consequent fall in vascular volume, is sensed by body sensors as a biochemical emergency. This kickstarts a sequence of actions.

Inhibitors of angiotensin converting enzyme are very successful blood pressure lowering medications widely used in clinical practice. This class of drugs are particularly preferred in treatment of high blood pressure seen in diabetic patients. New generation drugs targeting this biochemical axis include inhibitors of renin as well as inhibitors of angiotensin receptors. Even aldosterone antagonists are useful blood pressure lowering medications in a particular class of patients where there is overproduction of aldosterone in adrenal glands. I guess renin-angiotensin axis not only highlights the importance of finding suitable targets for achieving medical benefits but also illustrates the complexity of cell signalling itself.

One tidbit with regards to the Angiotensin converting enzyme II that is very valid now is the fact the COVID-19 virus uses this membrane-bound enzyme to gain illegal entry into the lung cells! Apparently, one of the viral membrane proteins called SPIKE resembles this angiotensin converting enzyme II! Intriguing! What on earth is angiotensin converting enzyme doing inside a lowly virus?

vii. Anaesthetic Drugs Work by Interfering with Nerve Impulse Conduction

Anaesthetic drugs act by preventing nerve impulses in sensory nerves thereby interfering with conduction of information about the pain. Basically, the information about pain (when the surgeon cuts your skin) is prevented from reaching the brain. How do we do that? The information about pain must be relayed by the pain receptors on the skin surface to the brain through neural conduction channels. If we interfere with this nerve conduction of information, then we can make the person unaware of the pain.

Local anaesthetics, which doctors use for minor surgical procedures like dental extraction etc. act by affecting the voltage-gated sodium channels in the nerve endings and by doing so these agents interfere with generation of nerve impulses by the pain receptors. You can also block major nerve roots, both sensory and motor conduction, by using certain anaesthetics that can be injected around the nerve plexus or peripheral nerve to be blocked. For example, epidural anaesthesia given during childbirth is one such regional anaesthetisation achieved by injecting anaesthetics into the lower back in the extradural space where it acts on the nerve roots. These agents help in interfering with the pain transmission through neural tracts.

General anaesthetics act on the brain, particularly on the Reticular Activating System (RAS). By acting on the GABA and glycine receptors (both inhibitory by nature) the general anaesthetics open the chloride channels that will make it difficult for generation of nerve impulses in the reticular activating system neurons. RAS consists of diffuse sensory nerve conduction fibres that relay vital sensory information to the brain.

These relay fibres are offshoots from main sensory information conduction tracts coming from the spinal cord when they join the base of the brain. The purpose of this RAS is to keep a person conscious. When the input into RAS is abolished, the brain loses the consciousness, which works fine for the surgeons. Sleep is a physiological state where RAS conduction is minimised. Coma is the extreme state where RAS conduction is long lasting and potentially irreversible. By interfering with the transmission of pain messages to the brain the person is made to go to 'sleep'. Whatever the surgeon is doing on your body with his surgical knives never reaches your brain. That means you do not feel the pain until the effect of the anaesthetic wears off.

In short, the anaesthetic doctors are hacking into your nerve impulse conduction particularly the pain information. The brain is duped.

Surgeons also want the muscles to be relaxed when they perform the operations. The anaesthetist helps here by using muscle relaxant drugs along with the anaesthetic agents. The muscle relaxants are also useful when patients are put on electroconvulsive therapy (shock treatment) when excessive muscular contraction can occur. These muscle relaxants work by typically blocking acetylcholine-mediated nerve impulse conduction to the muscles. Acetylcholine is the chemical message sent via the nerves to the muscles to initiate contraction. Neuromuscular blocking agents compete with acetylcholine at the signal transfer point.

Naturally occurring substances like toxins and venoms (e.g., botulinum toxin) can prevent the release of acetylcholine at the nerve endings. Drugs that act on the signal interface between nerve and the muscle can be completely paralysing to the extent even the muscles needed for breathing can be paralysed. This means that such patients need mechanical ventilation. The muscle relaxing agents work exactly like Curare, a naturally occurring poison. South American natives use the extract of a tree bark, from which curare can be obtained, to coat their arrows used for hunting. The natives are signal hackers without their knowledge.

The theme of information hacking continues.

viii. Drugs that are Aimed at the High Command

Our brain is the high command of our body. There are many different types of control centres inside the brain that control individual parts of the body or vital functions of the body. The nerve cells in the brain are the workforce of the brain. They need to be controlled first. Otherwise, there could be problems in the execution of the brain commands.

There are many types of brain diseases that can be traced back to deranged communication between nerve cells. Nerve cells communicate through electrical connections as much as they do use molecular messages called neurotransmitters.

Depression is a common psychiatric condition. It is said that in depression there is a deficiency of the neurotransmitters like noradrenaline and serotonin in the brain. The antidepressant medications prescribed by doctors rectify the situation by one of the 2 mechanisms: prevention of reuptake of these neurotransmitters at synapses (thereby prolonging the action of these neurotransmitters), or by inhibiting the enzyme (Monoamine oxidase) that degrades these neurotransmitters (again with the same effect of prolonged, sustained action of noradrenaline and serotonin). The best-selling antidepressant drug Prozac works by reuptake inhibition mechanism.

GABA is the most important inhibitory neurotransmitter in the brain. Just as stimulatory inputs are important it is even more important to bring some balance in neural signalling by having some form of inhibitory control. It is like your brake in the car. You cannot just have an accelerator to speed up. You also need the brake to slow down and stop. Brain cells cannot be left to speed away recklessly. You need to tame them.

GABA and glycine are well known inhibitory neurotransmitters whose job it is to silence nerve cells from firing away. Glutamate is a typical excitatory neurotransmitter. GABA-producing nerve cells are situated all over the brain and spinal cord but not outside these two structures. Interestingly, level of GABA stimulation or inhibition determines much of our brain's mental status and other higher neuronal functions. In the presence of more GABA activity (and therefore more inhibitory output in the brain) there is sedation, amnesia, muscle relaxation, lack of balance and coordination. Nervousness and anxiety are also reduced when GABA's inhibitory output increases which means that these emotions are mediated by stimulatory brain activity. GABA helps to control the feelings of anxiety and that is why pharmaceutical companies have targeted GABA receptor for developing drugs that can control anxiety.

Epilepsy is characterised by excessive neuronal discharges in the brain due to over excitability of the brain neurons. This can be due to localised or generalised hyper excitation of the brain. Medical treatment of epilepsy is aimed at calming the brain electrical activity. Drugs used for treatment of seizures are capable of stimulating GABA release in the brain. As GABA is primarily an inhibitory neurotransmitter this helps to lower brain neuronal discharges that fire signals to muscles indiscreetly. The effect is reduced muscular contraction and relief from the intense muscular contraction seen in many different types of seizures. Some of the drugs used for epilepsy also lower the stimulatory neurotransmitters like Glutamate. Some drugs like Vigabatrin and Valproate act by inhibiting the enzyme that degrades GABA prolonging the action of GABA at the GABA receptors. Drugs like Gabapentin are analogues of GABA itself so that they mimic GABA at the GABA receptor and bring about the same signal across the receptor.

As one can imagine many drugs used for neurological and psychiatric diseases are modulators/inhibitors/activators of neurotransmitter receptors. This is hardly surprising. Nerve-nerve communication and nerve-muscle communication are central to the function of the brain and the nervous system in our body.

ix. Getting the Better of our Invisible Enemies by Hitting Their Information Content

So far, we have been looking at cellular targets present in our own body that are medically manipulated to bring about a cure. We should not forget the fact that many of our diseases are brought on by microbes that infect our body. Such diseases caused by microbes are usually short-lived and, in many cases, self-limiting too.

This is true of many viral diseases such as common cold etc., but there are very serious infections that can be caused by many viruses like Ebola, AIDS, Marburg etc. In such serious forms of viral infection death can often result.

Bacterial infections are normally treated with antibiotics and there are quite a variety of antibiotics available in the doctor's armamentarium. With regards to the viruses, it is a sad truth that we do not have many effective treatments.

The point I want to bring up here is the fact the microbial diseases are treated by drugs that only attack the microbes. Ideally these drugs should leave the human cells alone. So, the molecular targets of drugs for infectious diseases are selectively targeted to the virus or bacteria.

Drugs that act against the bacteria work by 3 broad

mechanisms: inhibition of bacterial cell wall synthesis, inhibition of bacterial protein synthesis and inhibition of bacterial DNA synthesis. Commonly used antibiotics like Gentamycin, Tetracycline, Neomycin, Erythromycin etc. are information-hacking weapons really. They act by binding to bacterial ribosomes such that the bacterial protein synthesis is affected. Protein synthesis is the process whereby the nuclear code for the protein sequence is used for attaching individual amino acids in the right order. The binding of antibiotic to the ribosome interferes with this step and incorrect amino acids are attached. The protein that is formed is faulty and is unable to execute the required functions. The bacteria die. The mode of action of the antibiotics is information oriented. They prevent the ability of the bacteria to use their own genetic information to make executable molecular codes (namely proteins).

Antibiotics like Ciprofloxacin work differently. They inhibit bacterial (not human) Gyrase enzyme that is used by them for supercoiling the DNA. This supercoiling is needed to compact the DNA and without this the bacteria will not be able to undergo timely cell divisions. Bacterial multiplication is therefore avoided and helps us to curtail the growth and multiplication of the harmful microbes.

Co-trimoxazole contains two components: sulfamethoxazole inhibits dihydropteroate synthase and trimethoprim inhibits dihydrofolate reductase, essential for making DNA bases, an effect like some of the anticancer drugs. The result is the same. Without the bases the bacteria cannot make new DNA for the multiplying bacterial cells.

The most curious point we should not miss when we talk about antimicrobial drugs is the fact that many of them are derived from natural sources. We humans do not own the 'patent rights'. These drugs have been produced in the natural setting by competing life forms that use them as toxins to ward off competition in the ecological niche.

For example, a common source of antibacterial agents is the

fungus. The fungi produce antibiotic substances for the same reason we produce antibodies and cytokines within our immune system. For discussion of the topic in hand, it is more than interesting to note that bacterial warfare is also information-based! Modern medical science has conveniently adopted the microbial warfare tools!

Summary—All Drug Targets are Information-Related

I want to sum up finally—information is the very basis of survival in the animal kingdom. Without information transfer life systems cannot exist.

Curiously, we find that the motifs used for information handling by biological systems are so much like our own information technology and in many cases superior. The detailed description of all types of medicines used in the modern times clearly point to one single striking fact: they all act by interfering with information transfer of some sort.

There is no exception.

This vindicates my argument that human diseases are the result of failure or altered information exchange between cells. But I have shown in the two previous chapters how all human diseases can be brought within Shannon's information theory framework. Now I present irrefutable evidence from the pharmaceutical industry that all medicines work some way or other modulating or interfering with cellular information flow.

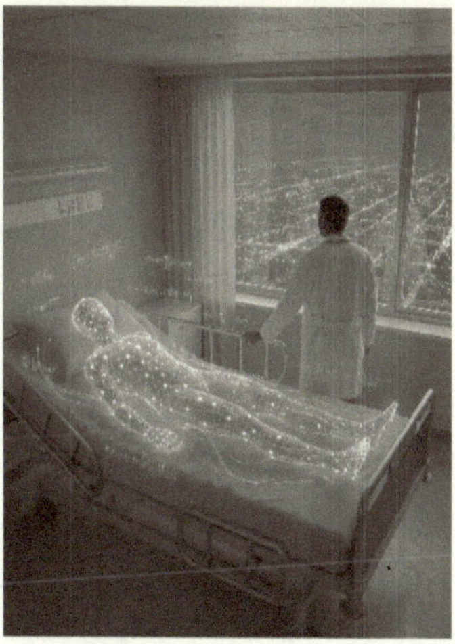

14. Final Common Pathway to Death

DOCTORS, ESPECIALLY THOSE practising acute medicine, know only too well that patients admitted for various illnesses, often progress through a strikingly similar course in the end. This phenomenon has been described as the 'final common pathway of disease and death'. What the above phenomena indicates is that there is convergence in disease pathways despite the diversity in aetiology. This interesting fact has not been explored adequately in the medical literature. This chapter aims to unravel the underlying mechanisms of this convergence.

In simple words one could say that when a person suffers from a disease the destination is always death. People may begin the journey from different starting points. But at some point, the journey starts converging into a single highway that takes you to the 'City of Death'. There is a saying 'all roads lead to Rome'. I guess in medical parlance we can revise this saying as 'all diseases lead to death'. May be some roads could be small, narrow roads and so could take a longer time to reach the destination. I suppose this is like the chronic, non-acute type of diseases that is not a fast superhighway to death. In some cases, the disease is acute and can take you swiftly to your destination in no time.

The point I am trying to drive home is that whatever roads you began your journey on will not matter after some point. All these roads will begin to converge on a small set of roads which will eventually end up in one final route. This is the final common pathway.

The primary aetiological agent and the pathogenic mechanism(s) of the primary disease of a dying patient could have been one of hundreds of known causes of disease in man but, after the initial insult to the system through biological, physical or chemical agents, which resulted in a disease, the subsequent course of events in most if not all diseases are surprisingly not specific to the disease at all. This is true in both acute and non-acute illnesses. This is truly a remarkable finding in medical practice that might have surprised most doctors, especially those who practise acute medicine.

Doctors know that for every symptom there are several differential diagnoses. This simply means that a symptom can be produced by many different diseases. The correct diagnosis is only made by looking for some diagnostic features that throw light on the aetiology (which still does not change the clinical manifestations suffered by the patient). Though the clinical consequences are identical the doctors need to know the aetiology in order to be able to treat the underlying cause.

For example, a patient could have anaemia due to tens of causes. It could arise due to iron deficiency, blood loss, haemolysis, bone marrow disorders, thalassemia, malaria, chronic diseases like cancer, renal failure etc. and so on but the clinical/biochemical effects of anaemia on the human body, and the courses of events due to these effects, are indistinguishable. It is true that they will have some diagnostic features that will help differentiate the cause of anaemia, but all anaemic patients will suffer the same types of clinical consequences of anoxia, and it does not matter whether he or she became anaemic due to blood loss or iron deficiency or bone marrow disorders.

Interestingly, adrenal insufficiency can arise due to a variety of aetiological factors (destruction of the adrenal gland by tuberculosis, autoimmune disorders, histiocytosis X, adrenoleukodystrophy, amyloidosis, sarcoidosis, histoplasmosis, adrenal haemorrhage, infarction etc.) and the biochemical outcome of the adrenal gland failure will be the same irrespective of the diverse aetiologies mentioned above.

Cardiac arrhythmias can be caused by myocardial factors like ischemia, infarction and myocarditis, autonomic imbalance like sympathetic and parasympathetic over-activity/ under-activity, Electrolyte imbalance like hypokalemia and hypomagnesemia Hypoxia, Drugs like antiarrhythmic agents and psychotropic agents,

Genetic disorders like Channelopathies like Brugada syndrome, long QT syndrome and short QT syndrome but the outcome of disorderly beating of the heart is reduced or absent cardiac output, fall in blood pressure and low oxygenation in tissues.

Hypopituitarism can be caused by tumors compressing the pituitary gland, infections within brain like encephalitis, meningitis, hemochromatosis, autoimmune hypophysitis, pituitary apoplexy, physical causes like brain injury, surgery and ionizing radiations or congenital factors. The outcome of hypopituitarism is the same.

What really happens is that the various biological and physical insults that triggered the disease phenomenon in an organ will invariably produce effects that seem to converge on progressively decreasing number of pathways like a funnel effect.

Then there is further narrowing of the outcomes to one or two critical pathways and because these critically important pathways govern global processes the effect of this funneling leads to widespread breakdown of the life processes simultaneously. At this stage it does not matter what were the initial disease-triggering causes at all. They lose their identity and what matters is the biological and physical changes they brought about.

It is probably easier to understand this by looking at a real-world example.

Famine is a mass killer that can wipe out an entire population. Famine is absence of food. Absence of food can be caused by failed crops. The crops can fail due to diseases of the plants or lack of water or due to pests or due to land degradation.

It does not matter what was the original cause as the result will be the same - famine.

Transport problems due to lack of fuel or lack of drivers or lack of roads or lack of carriers can also affect the food distribution creating the same effects caused by failed agriculture. In the modern days the supermarkets can be found to become very quickly empty for flimsy reasons like lack of drivers of lorries!

We are as vulnerable as that.

International relations and border restrictions can again cause food shortages very soon as foods these days travel long distances to reach their consumers. Lack of jobs, and lowered or absent buying capacity of people, can cause the same effect of non-availability of food and it does not matter at that stage whether agriculture flourished or there were no faults in logistics of food distribution. Or prices of foods can skyrocket, and people cannot simply afford to buy them.

One can cite many causes, local or widespread, that can cause shortage or absence of food in a society. It matters little what triggered it. The result will be starvation and death. All the diverse causes culminate in one final endpoint i.e., lack of food energy. The lack of food energy has far-reaching, remote effects that will cause deaths of millions.

Famine and poverty are words that apply to society. Hunger and malnutrition are equivalent terms at the individual level. Cells starve during times of malnutrition.

Whatever the cause of malnutrition is the effects will be the same. That is the point.

i. What Determines the Acute vs. Chronic Course of the Disease?

We know that diseases can be acute or chronic in onset. We also know that some diseases lead to death while others cause only morbidity.

Death-causing diseases can also differ in the time frame needed to produce death. A myocardial infarction patient will die in minutes whereas a cancer patient will do so in months to years. Again, some chronic diseases like, for example, diabetes mellitus, can lead to life-threatening states such as diabetic ketoacidosis, even though the well-managed diabetic patient can survive very long without an immediate threat to his or her life.

What determines the differences in the nature of the diseases?

I argue that a disease that affects a key biochemical or cellular pathway is likely to lead to acute changes.

This is because effects on critical biochemical pathways are likely to have far-reaching, remote effects on the body. On the contrary, non-acute diseases only produce effects at the local tissue or organ level only. An arthritis patient is not likely to face a life-threatening, sudden progression of disease because joint degradation is not going to compromise a critical cellular or molecular event.

Of course, the bone and synovial epithelial cells do get affected but these effects are going to be localised.

So, the other useful way of distinguishing an acute from a chronic disease is by looking for global effects of the disease process i.e., wide-ranging effects on multiple or all cell types, as opposed to localised cellular effects as we see in diseases such as arthritis or skin disorders etc.

ii. What are the Critical Biochemical Pathways that have Global Effects?

To help understand the concept we can look at our everyday life. In your routine life you do different kinds of activities. It could be part of your job or your household responsibilities. Just sit for a moment and think. What are those things that you can just brush aside and carry on without much worry? What are those things that will impact on your overall financial well-being or health or your family life? What are the things that will impact over a short term only? What are the things that are likely to last for a long time? What are the things that will finish you off?

Our body is just like that. It is a conglomerate of trillions of cells working together. Hundreds of cellular processes happen daily inside our body. Not all of them have the same impact on survival. There are some processes that will have a direct and immediate impact on survival. This is because these processes will affect multiple tissues and organs (global effects). On the contrary, there are some processes that will affect only one or two tissues and therefore have a localised effect only. They do not impact on survival but may cause some degree of discomfort. This may show in the form of some minor to moderate illness.

What are the biochemical processes that will have global, far-reaching effects inside the body? Surely, one can think of oxygen levels. If ever there was a problem in oxygenation, either due to lung diseases or heart diseases, the low oxygen level (hypoxia) or total lack of oxygen level (anoxia) will affect every single cell in the body. It is like lack of fuel for our cars, lack of electricity for our factories, lack of food for our bodies.

I suppose one can think of low blood volume as another situation where all cells are likely to be impacted. Low blood volume can happen due to serious blood loss, dehydration, etc. Low blood pressure can result due to this which will affect the ability of the heart to pump food fuel and nutrients all around.

Several entities/constituents in the human body are tightly

regulated because they are critically important for life-sustaining processes. For example, oxygen, sodium, potassium, calcium, phosphate, glucose, water, magnesium, hydrogen ions, nutrients, blood volume, blood pressure, carbon di oxide, osmolality, etc. are maintained within normal limits all the time. The concentrations of important constituents, be they elements or nutrients, fluctuate under normal circumstances but they are 'attracted' to the central point by the regulatory influences.

These 'attractors' are the regulatory agents/cellular mechanisms like relevant hormones and neurotransmitters, which themselves are subjected to lots of feedback and feed-forward controls. In fact, every process or constituent operates within almost a rigid limit. The rigidity is less when the process or constituent is not critical. In order to define what this 'criticality' is I prefer the simple test—Is the effect produced local or global? Agents or processes that produce global effects within the body are likely to be far more tightly controlled.

There are a few adaptive mechanisms that kick in when there are deviations from the central point and life is sustainable when these deviations fall within a certain limit.

Sodium and Potassium salts are important for our body to function. Not having enough sodium or potassium or chloride is like have a battery that has depleted salt levels inside. It will not work.

There are many other minerals of importance in our body. They are calcium, phosphorus, nitrogen, magnesium etc. They play crucial roles in many different biochemical and physiological processes. For those of you wondering why minerals should be so important they are well advised to follow news reports around the world. Countries are ready to go to war to seek minerals and rare earth elements like Lithium, Cobalt, manganese, nickel, silicon, aluminium, copper, silver, tungsten etc. Because these minerals are needed for a variety of industries. The same applies to our body. The minerals needed for our body are to be sourced at all costs.

Sodium and potassium concentrations in the blood and extra

cellular fluid are vital for the cells because they help in neural transmissions. In other words, all the communications between nerve cells, muscle cells and the sensory receptors depend on sodium and potassium. They maintain the right electrical environment inside the cells for them to activate or shut down electrical signals. The flipping of the negative interior to positive and the reversal mimics the on/off (0/1) kind of switching that we see in transistors. Basically, the sodium, potassium elements, by virtue of their movement across the cell reversibly change the electrical charge from negative to positive and then back to negative. This reversible switching helps create the potential for information coding like we see in chips.

Sodium-potassium pump determines the negative cellular interior (-50 to 70 mV) and generation of the action potentials and is the very basis of all cellular communication between neurons and neuromuscular transmission that we see in motor coordination, generation of intrinsic excitation of cardiac cells (the basis of cardiac rhythm), action potentials in sensory receptors determining information capture (vision, hearing, touch etc.), intrinsic rhythms in neuronal groups such as the supremely important respiratory centre in the brain etc.

In other words, these electrolytes determine the excitability of cells, the very hallmark of living systems. Because of the nature of the roles played by these two electrolytes the outcomes of any disorders in their regulation will have a global effect on the body.

Doctors who have treated conditions like hyponatremia/hypernatremia (low and high Sodium concentration in the blood) and hypokalaemia/hyperkalaemia (low and high potassium concentration in the blood) only know too well how devastating these conditions can be.

Complexity of adaptive responses to restore constancy of these critical parameters is illustrated in the figure which depicts the sequence of events that would happen, for example, when there is a fall in sodium concentration in the extra cellular fluid. Smooth muscle cells in the arterial walls constrict, intestinal cells activate salt and water reabsorption and neural centres in hypothalamus trigger thirst and salt appetite work and their collective actions lead to a common goal of expansion of blood volume and an efficient circulation.

Diseases of the adrenal gland, especially adrenal insufficiency, can lead to a deficiency of this aldosterone and cortisol, another hormone concerned with sodium homeostasis produced by adrenal gland, and therefore could interfere with our ability to maintain the constancy of the sodium concentration.

That means that diseases affecting some vital organs and glands can lead to interference in the remedial mechanisms that aim to restore the balance.

Let me give an example. Our blood volume is about 5 litres. Blood is constantly pumped around by the action of the heart. The heart is literally a motor. It is vitally important that the blood volume is kept tightly controlled. Otherwise, the effect is the same as what would happen if a river started drying out. Transportation of essential goods becomes difficult. Nutrients and oxygen cannot be supplied to all the cells. This is a grave threat to the body. Immediately, restoration mechanisms are kick-started. This is the essence of what a physiologist would call 'Homeostasis'. It is about maintaining key essential parameters within a tightly controlled narrow range. Fluctuations are OK but they are never allowed to cross critical cut off levels.

Going back to our example of low blood volume let us see what happens. Our body is a well-equipped cybernetic system. It has receptors that can pick up falling blood volume and pressure. They are molecular receptors that can sense the vascular pressure as well as the vascular volume. Pressure receptors (also called baroreceptors) are situated on the walls of arteries, atrial chamber of the heart and kidneys. They will start firing when the blood volume starts falling. There are also receptors that can sense the volume. These receptors are situated within the thoracic cavity. Both pressure receptors and volume receptors send input to the Juxtaglomerular cells in the kidney to start secreting Angiotensin, a versatile molecule that can play a critical role in restoration of the blood volume.

Firstly, Angiotensin acts on the heart muscle cells to pump faster and stronger to help improve the blood flow. Angiotensin also acts on the hypothalamus to stimulate thirst and appetite for salt. As one can imagine drinking more fluids and consuming more salt replenishes the blood volume.

Angiotensin must act through a molecular receptor that can decode the signal carried by Angiotensin. Adrenal gland cells have the receptor for Angiotensin. In response to Angiotensin the adrenal gland secretes Aldosterone which, in turn, starts retaining sodium from the glomerular filtrate. Otherwise, this sodium would be excreted as waste in urine. By retaining sodium, the body also retains more water due to the osmotic pull of sodium. The final effect is expansion of the blood volume.

As one can see, so many cells work together to bring about a concerted action towards a common goal. We are hardly aware of what is going on behind the scenes. These biochemical actions never reach the conscious space. Communication and sharing of information are central to cellular cooperation. What would happen if the baroreceptor and volume receptor cells are unable to pick out the signals properly? What would happen of the kidneys are diseased such that they do not respond to the baroreceptor signals which means that there will be no Angiotensin. What would happen if the adrenal gland cells do not respond to signals coming in the form of Angiotensin? There will be no secretion of Aldosterone and no retention of sodium and water.

This is what I am trying to convey. Cells need to communicate. When there is a lapse in this communication there is disease.

Let us move on with other vital parameters essential for continuation of life. It is impossible to overemphasise the importance of oxygen in life. Oxygen is vital in this process of life because it is needed to burn your food 'fuel' to release the energy which is no different from the way our fossil fuels depend on oxygen to combust them! This happens inside the cellular power factories called the mitochondria. These powerhouses make the adenosine triphosphate (ATP), the cellular energy currency. Oxygen is the fuel for our body to burn our food and generate energy. About 3 or 4 minutes of anoxia can irreversibly damage brain neurons and can cause brain death. Heart muscles will cease their pumping within this timeframe. Lack of energy will shut down the membrane pumps and the metabolic pathways. All cellular constituents irrevocably move towards a state of equilibrium, colloquially referred to as death. So, the numerous initial triggers that compromise oxygen availability in the body, which come under respiratory and heart diseases category, culminate in a one-way path towards the state of death.

Other factors like minerals such as magnesium, calcium and phosphate are also crucial in cell survival each one of them having their own parts to play. Because phosphate is needed in synthesis of ATP and magnesium is needed because it is a co-factor for enzymes that use ATP any diseases that lead to deficiencies in these parameters will have global consequences however localised the initial disruptions were. Calcium is important too in muscle-neuron communication as calcium initiates the muscle contraction. Calcium is also extremely important in cellular communication, apart from its role in muscular contraction, as the most important 'tertiary messenger' for a variety of messengers. Phosphate is also critical in acid-base balance and, more importantly, in regulation of intermediary metabolism and cell signalling. Enzymes and informational second messengers can be covalently modified by addition (through kinases) and by removal (through phosphatases) of phosphate groups. Such phosphorylation/dephosphorylation is a ubiquitous mechanism in control of cellular information flow.

Without going too much in detail it will suffice to say that there are a few other critical parameters like water content, osmolality, glucose, blood pressure and volume etc. which tend to have far-reaching, global effects on the body when things go out of control. We may not find such far-reaching global effects for every constituent in the body. There is a difference in criticality.

To use a simple example for the sake of illustrating the concept just sit back and think for a while what are those things in your life that are indispensable, and what are those things that will make it difficult to live, and what are those things that you would not even care about. This will make you understand the concept. I am pretty sure your analysis will show that there are a few items in your life that will make it impossible to carry on living. Whereas there will be a few will have major impact, but you can still plod on. There will be a few items which really do not matter. They will be like mosquito-bites and nothing more.

iii. Final Common Pathway of Disease and Death: Could Convergence of Diverse Disease Processes on Key Biochemical Processes be the Explanation?

A striking feature of human diseases is that the innumerable forms of disease-causing insults like physical agents (heat, radiation etc.), biological systems (microbes), chemical (poisons, drugs etc.), biochemical disturbances (hormonal deficiencies and excesses) or genetic factors (DNA damage) will produce convergent biochemical effects affecting one or more of the vital homeostatic processes such as ones mentioned above. There are a convergence of diverse aetiological factors leading to common biochemical outcomes that can potentially lead to global effects within the multicellular life system.

Firstly, let us list the most important biochemical parameters that need to be absolutely kept within a tightly controlled range failing which there is a direct threat to continuation of life.

This list should include:

- low or high blood sodium,
- low of high blood potassium

- low of high blood pressure and volume
- low levels of oxygen
- Too acidic or alkaline blood
- High carbon di oxide levels in blood
- Low or high calcium levels in blood
- Low or high magnesium levels in blood
- Low or high phosphate levels in blood
- Low or high glucose level in blood
- Low or high body temperature

The parameters listed above are critically important ones that need to be tightly controlled within a narrow range. If allowed to stary too high or too low these parameters can start posing a risk to continuation of life. The most striking feature of perturbations in these parameters is that the effects are global. In other words, the effects are far reaching and likely to affect the entire body. The effects are not going to be localized to single tissue or organ. That is what needs to be considered when we talk about the final common pathway to death.

It is not difficult to understand the far reaching effects of anoxia, low levels of oxygen in the blood. Virtually, all cells in the body will be affected. Without oxygen there is no combustion of food. Without food combustion there is no energy generation (ATP) inside the cells. All cells will grind to a halt.

Too low or high sodium or potassium levels will start interfering with the excitability of cells (muscular, neural and all). Because the cell's ability to initiate action potential will be hampered. The word 'action potential' refers to the change from the electronegative cellular interior to a reversible electro positivity. This is the basis of all cellular conduction and excitation, the very hallmark of the living state. It is what makes the cells alive and responsive. By interfering with this ability drastic changes on sodium and potassium levels would lead to global unresponsiveness of cells, consistent with death.

Severe alterations in blood volume will lead to catastrophic logistic issues in supply of oxygen and nutrients to all cells.

Gross changes in calcium, Magnesium and hydrogen ions will affect neuromuscular function globally.

Changes in acid-base balance will have wide impact on metabolic reactions as all our metabolic enzymes are designed to work well at a pH of 7.4. Too high or low hydrogen ions will shift the pH away from the optimum range needed for proper enzymic functions. The same applies to changes in body temperature. Our cellular enzymes need an optimum body temperature of 37 degrees Celsius. This is all about enzyme kinetics. Our cells are bags of enzymes, aren't they? Someone who fell in freezing water or ice would begin to have a shutdown of all cellular enzymes and there is no metabolism possible to sustain life.

Too low glucose level in our blood would have the same effect as our machines that ran out of fuel or power. No cell will be spared.

What is to be noted is that perturbations in the above parameters can be caused by various factors that seem to have a converging effect.

For instance, polyuria due to hypothalamic disease (infection, infarction, tumour, infiltration) causing a defect in release of Antidiuretic hormone, Nephrogenic Diabetes Insipidus, impairment of thirst mechanism (coma, confusion, immobility) can all lead to dehydration and high sodium levels in the body. All these diverse aetiologies seem to converge on one of the global, life-sustaining pathways. This is figuratively like a journey you undertake trying to reach a destination. There may be many roads you can take to reach your destination but at some point, your options are going to be fewer as you near a destination. It is exactly like 'All roads lead to Rome'.

Let us see another example of a global perturbation. Let us look at low sodium levels in blood. Adrenal failure, extra-renal loss (Gastrointestinal loss, burns, haemorrhage), dilutional effects of water retention states (oedema), syndrome of inappropriate antidiuretic hormone secretion (lung infections, lung cancer, drugs etc) and finally renal loss of sodium can all lead to low sodium levels (hyponatremia).

Decreased dietary uptake, Gastrointestinal loss (fistula, diarrhoea), increased intracellular uptake, renal loss due to aldosterone overactivity, and different conditions that cause renal tubular damage and consequent leakage of potassium in the urine can all lead to low levels of blood potassium (hypokalaemia).

Lysis of cells and release of cellular potassium and decreased renal excretion due to aldosterone underactivity, renal failure and drugs such as diuretics can cause high potassium levels in blood (hyperkalaemia).

Both hypo- and hyperkalaemia are immediately life-threatening. The initial causes of these life-threatening perturbations can be many and varied. But they all converge on a final common pathway.

Respiratory diseases (obstructive and infiltrative), diseases of the central nervous system such as damage to the base of the brain affecting the respiratory centre, nerve damage to phrenic nerve innervating the diaphragm, thoracic diseases like cage deformities or diaphragmatic diseases, circulatory defects (hypovolemia, anaemia, cardiac failure etc) can all converge of oxygen levels in the body.

This is like the most final common pathway. All 'disease roads' leading to death will at some point converge of the oxygen road. All patients who die in emergency wards or intensive care wards may have been admitted for various ailments. But when they die the death punch was from lack of oxygen. This is the killer blow. Mortality data published by WHO shows that majority of the deaths occur worldwide due to diseases of the respiratory and cardiovascular system, and one can see why. Because these diseases that converge on oxygen availability.

Decreased food intake, due to disease or poverty, Gastrointestinal absorption defects, insulin secreting tumours, underacting thyroid, underacting pituitary, glycogen storage diseases, disorders of gluconeogenesis, liver disease etc can all lead to hypoglycaemia, a condition where there is a shortage of glucose in the blood. This condition can be fatal if unattended. The brain will shut down when glucose level falls below 35 mg per decilitre just as your mobile devices run out of power.

Be warned that the brain shut down is irreversible.

It is not as if you can recharge your brain back to power.

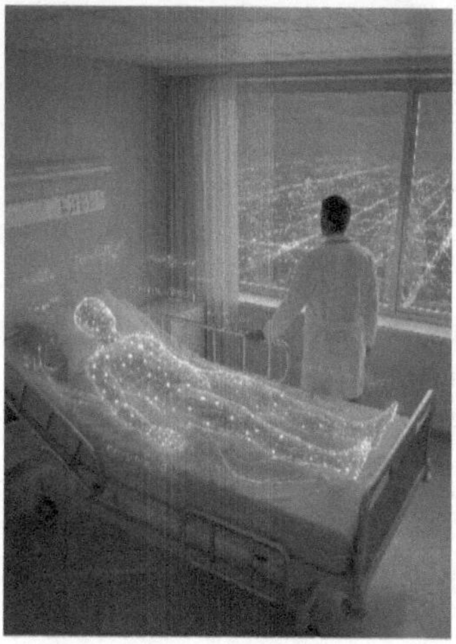

15. Information Failure as the Basis of all Human Diseases

THERE ARE MANY trillion cells inside our body. It is obvious that they need to exchange information between each other to know who is doing what. In your outside world you may have the newspapers, news channels, Radio, mobile phones etc. that help you to gather information while at the same time send information. But what do the cells inside your body have? Is it even conceivable that they just go about doing their functions the way they like? Or, at any time they like?

Individual cells inside our body are functionally and structurally discrete units. In every sense of the word, they are citizens of the body by right of birth. They are duty-bound' to the welfare of the body. No wonder they work in unison with other fellow cellular citizens. That is the way complex systems behave. Cooperation is at the heart of complex systems. If cells must cooperate, they need to 'know'.

Information is now believed to be a fundamental property of matter in the universe. It plays a primal role in the way systems work. Invariably, all our social transactions are based on some form of information transfer or other. It is presumable that any multi-unit system will depend on information exchange between the individual components that constitute it. Claude Shannon, in his seminal paper in 1948, defined information as 'a reduction in the uncertainty' and formulated a mathematical theory for communication. The reduction in the uncertainty refers to the gain in the information about an entity, brought about by reproducing at one point either exactly or approximately a message selected at another point.

Basically, a typical communication system, as described by Shannon, consists of a message source, a coder to encrypt the information, a channel for communication, and finally a decoder to receive the information. His information theory was developed to understand the transmission of electronic signals. But this theory now has had an impact on biology as well, particularly with reference to DNA, because of the obvious relationship between DNA and biological information.

It is amazing to see that the intercellular communication happens like a relay race. From the message source (such as DNA) coded, information-rich molecules are generated and released.

Examples of such information codes include hormones, neurotransmitters, growth factors etc. These informational molecules are carried in blood stream or neural pathways which are the channels of communication in Shannon terms.

Once the molecular primary codes reach their respective cellular destinations they are received by cell-surface, molecular aerials called receptors. Each type of primary informational messenger will find a unique, specific molecular receptor on their target cells. These specific receptors alone will have the ability to decode the primary message. Subsequent information relay would involve secondary messengers (such as cyclic AMP) generated by these cell-surface receptors. They carry the information deep inside the cell to effector molecules. In many cases, there may be a further round of information relay involving a tertiary (third) messenger (such as Calcium). The final effect would be brought about by the direct action of the third messenger on the required intracellular structure.

The beauty of this set up is that the whole sequence of message transfer is set in stone. It has happened this way for ages. Cells have an established protocol for communicating with each other through this information relay.

There is a paucity of research looking at information transfer between and within cells through processes distal to the DNA. There has been virtually no effort to view the body, made up of tens of trillions of cells, as a 'cellular society' reliant on information exchange between cells to function. Presumably, unlike DNA and protein sequences lending themselves to study of the principles of encoding and information content, the 'communication channels' in intercellular exchange of information and the mechanisms of decoding are not amenable to mathematical studies.

The 'communication channels' in organisms include obviously the nerves but abundant amount of information transfer occurs in biological systems through non-neural routes through the agency of information-rich molecules which are secreted by endocrine, paracrine and autocrine systems.

Information can be 'packed' in biochemical molecules by a series of well-regulated steps. Messages coming from a source are encoded by certain types of cells and the encoded message is transmitted via the blood stream or the nerves. The decoders are usually receptor molecules stationed at the outer surface of the cell. The receiver cell responds to these molecular messages with an appropriate biological response.

I believe that huge multicellular organisms are vulnerable to cellular disorder and humans are no exception. The human body is estimated to contain tens of trillions of cells, which perform tasks according to their structural and functional specialisation. They function as one whole because they are inter-linked by a communication network the complexity of which is mind-boggling and still not completely understood.

Information transfer is central to the process of metabolic control and cells constantly exchange information with regards to fuel levels, blood pressure, nutrient concentrations, oxygen, minerals like sodium, potassium, calcium, phosphate, magnesium etc. and any deviation in the internal environment is attended by compensatory mechanisms that will restore the constancy. Invariably, these adaptive mechanisms require a chain of communication between effectors and target cells, often involving several cell types.

Physical, biological or chemical insults can lead to difficulties in cellular communication which can be localised to a particular organ or to a limited number of cell types, or can be widespread affecting multiple or, where death is imminent, all cell types. The resultant phenomenon is disease. Death is the final state in the evolution of the disease where the coherent functioning of all cells is no longer feasible due to global information failure. When the adaptive mechanisms of homeostasis fail, due to failure of one or more cell types to either generate or respond to informational molecules, the outcome is a disorderly state that is not responsive to the internal nor the external environment of the body.

I call this state as disease and the body as a system will manifest biochemical and clinical features that are diagnostic.

That is why I feel that the phenomenon of disease should be unique to only multi-cellular life forms, and not unicellular life. For that matter, even (natural) death should be a unique multi-cellular life property. Unicellular microbes endlessly divide into daughter cells in the presence of adequate nutrient supply and so do cancer cells, which behave autonomously much like unicellular life.

Every homeostatic process in the human body, as said above, is achieved by hormonal and/or neuro-endocrine mechanisms through release of specific informational molecules. The sources of this information are the regulatory cells like endocrine glands and neural control centres like hypothalamus. These information generating cells themselves depend on information coming in the form of internal feedback from target cells or external information from the sensory organs. It is a two-way communication.

An incredible amount of information capture (from the external world) and transmission (to neural processing centres and onto effecter cells) occurs in our body relating to acquisition of nutrients, identification of the enemy or predator (for self-protection), and a reproductive mate (for propagating the genes). Practically all our energy and cellular capabilities are directed towards physical work to fulfil these functions.

To carry out these biological roles the cells need to communicate between them, in terms of exchange of information about the current body situation, and whether the internal environment has the optimum chemical composition to prepare the body for work towards fulfilment of these functions. Any disturbance in the communication networks of body cells would lead to a breakdown of the adaptive mechanisms resulting in biochemical/systemic manifestations as said above. These biochemical disturbances, such as low oxygen availability, or low sodium, potassium, calcium or phosphate concentrations, which arise due to defective cell communication between selected cell types, could have a further cascading effect leading to global effects on information transfer, which is the forerunner of death.

In this chapter I have avoided as much medical terminology as possible and tried to convey the ideas in a simplified manner. Some would find it still hard to digest but I hope that those readers may have to try a bit harder.

I have explored the concept of disease from a biological perspective viewing it as a failure to maintain the constancy of the internal environment of the body due to defects in intercellular communication. I have shown that diverse disease-causing mechanisms produce convergent effects on key biochemical processes to bring about global disruption in the communication capabilities of the cells. I have attempted to show that multi-cellular life systems like humans, consisting of trillions of cells, are vulnerable to cellular disorder as a result of this breakdown of information transfer resulting in an inability to function as a cohesive unit. In summary, I claim that the information failure is the basis of cellular disorder associated with all human diseases.

When the adaptive mechanisms of homeostasis fail, due to failure of one or more cell types to either generate or respond to informational molecules, the outcome is a disorderly state that is not responsive to the internal or the external environment of the body. I call this state as disease and the body as a system will manifest biochemical and clinical features that are diagnostic.

Physical, biological or chemical insults can lead to difficulties in cellular communication which can be localised to a particular organ or to a limited number of cell types, or can be widespread affecting multiple or, where death is imminent, all cell types. The resultant phenomenon is disease. Death is the final state in the evolution of the disease where the coherent functioning of all cells is no longer feasible due to global information failure.

The primary reason why maintenance of the constancy of the internal environment is so crucial to the property of life in multicellular life forms is the absolute necessity of a localised and unique internal milieu that is distinguishable from the vast and changing external environment to fulfil the definition of a life system. In a philosophical sense, it is necessary for differentiating between 'self' and 'non-self' and in a biological sense this is needed to create an ideal composition of the fluids with the right amounts of life-supporting elements creating a conducive environment for life processes.

The internal body fluids of a human being, as well as any other multicellular life form, have optimum concentrations of sodium, potassium, calcium, magnesium, phosphate, hydrogen ions, oxygen, carbon di oxide, water, fuels, other nutrients like vitamins, trace elements etc. These compounds and minerals are available in the external environment, but they are not present in a circumscribed space, and, in addition, their concentrations fluctuate quite widely and, most of all, may not be readily available in a useable form, which are unfavourable features for sustenance of life.

Why do we have a kitchen? Why do we have restaurants?

Because these are the places where we have accumulated life-sustaining food items for our use. The items that we keep in the kitchen, or the restaurant, did not grow there. They are available in nature. They are grown in farms dotted all over the country or even other countries from where they were imported. They may be found in forests. They may be growing in the mountains. But you cannot go to a mountain or a forest or another country every time you need food. You cannot go searching for a river every time you need to drink.

Do you get the point?

Life systems 'create' a kitchen inside every cell where all required elements are available in the right quantities and at the right times. That is what maintenance of constancy of internal environment is all about. When your stock levels are going down you top them up by going to a grocery shop. We make regular weekly visits to the grocer because we know the consumption patterns of food items. Yet, we still must make occasional top up visits to the nearby shop for things like milk or bread.

Imagine a situation when your local grocery shop runs out of some items. You will go to another nearby shop. If not some supermarket near or far. You will try to place orders online if necessary. Some people living in the countryside may grow their own food. What is important is maintaining a steady level of food supplies in your kitchen. Without knowing we are performing the 'homeostatic' balance just like what your internal body cells do.

Any deviation in the body's internal environment is attended by compensatory mechanisms that will restore the constancy. If the compensatory mechanisms fail, then a stage is reached where there is equilibration of contents of the internal and external environment of your body. We colloquially call this state as death.

In other words, life is possible only if the distinction between the external and internal environment can be maintained at the expense of considerable energy. Failing this, the distinction disappears, and the principles of chemical equilibrium set in, dissolving the barrier between you as a life system and the vast expanses of the rest of the world!

Going back to the analogy of the household and the kitchen inside it, if you run out of food in your kitchen then your house becomes unsuitable for living. The contents inside the house are no different from the street outside completely devoid of life-sustaining food. You failed to maintain the constancy of the internal environment of the house endangering the sustenance of life. Some readers may think of ordering food online or go to a restaurant. Or even go hunting.

These measures will only work for a period.

When all households face the same situation of shortage of food even online suppliers and restaurants will find their internal contents disappear. Their internal environment will cease to be distinguishable from the streets outside, a state not conducive to living.

History is replete with instances when famine hits the nations, and millions die. I suppose I can call the famine as a failed homeostasis at the societal level. Failed crops due to disease, or drought or even poverty can all contribute to this sordid situation.

I said communication is vital for body cells to source all the vital ingredients from incoming supplies i.e., eating and drinking. Hunger centre in the brain and the thirst centre, basically sensors made up of nerve cells, initiate the 'import' of food and water respectively when there is a shortage of goods.

How can they do it if they are not told when and how much?

The food raw materials are used to make 'value-added molecular goods' that are required by cells. They need to know when to make what. Just for a moment imagine a scenario where our global businesses are run without any information tools. If you do not have phones or faxes or emails between people and between companies the global supply of goods will grind to a halt making people run from pillar to post for their essentials. Or, on the contrary, the factories may end up with a glut. The businesses needlessly manufactured too much of the goods and there are no takers.

It is difficult to refute the argument that information exchange between cells is as vital as in our business world. The word 'logistics' has become firmly established in the modern-day world as the centre of our modern-day existence. Cellular logistics is even more complex and coordinated than ours and that requires communication between cells. The cellular communication networks can go awry under certain situations, and they will have consequences. The severity can be minor to major. I am now attempting to show that these information failures are the sources of human diseases which is a viewpoint not hitherto put forward in any standard medical texts.

I have shown below the kinds of errors that can creep into the cellular communication networks. Earlier I alluded to the point that the biological information exchange can come under the principle of Claude Shannon's Information theory. Based on the concept of Shannon's model, it can be deduced that errors in information transmission within the human body can occur due to Defects in information source, Coding, transmission and channel errors and Decoding (Receiver) errors.

I elaborate this with a brief explanation for each category with examples to illustrate the point.

A. Defects in Information Sources

THERE ARE AT least 3 fundamental sources of information in the human body, and perhaps all animals. They are namely DNA, the heart and the brain.

In the case of DNA, it is obvious. DNA is the blueprint of life. We will come back to the relation between defects in DNA information and the origin of human disease a bit later after we have discussed the heart and brain first.

I. The Heart as a Rhythmic Electrical Signal Generator

The heart is an electrically operated motor. This motor continues to work non-stop from the time you were in your mother's womb to the time you settle down comfortably in your grave. If it stops, you stop living. The primary driver is the intrinsic electrical stimulus generated within the heart itself. The sino-atrial node, a patch of specialised heart tissue, located within the atrium, is the supreme site where the heart impulses are repetitively generated about 72 times a minute.

Without any external input the cells here automatically fire, spreading this electrical impulse down a pre-determined conduction pathway to reach every nook and corner of the heart. It is this autonomously generated electrical signal that unifies the pumping action of all heart muscle fibres. This rhythmic signal is at the centre of life itself because if this signal does not come then the heart stops beating and within 3 or 4 minutes all life activities will grind to a halt. It is amazing nature has evolved such a brilliant, automated process to ensure non-stop beating of the heart.

Amazingly, if you isolate a single heart muscle cell (not the whole heart) it can be shown to beat repetitively. That is, it contracts repetitively which you can see under the microscope. For this the isolated cell should be placed in a salt solution.

If you put a number of these isolated heart muscle cells together in solution then amazingly, all of them will start beating in unison!

This is because the cells start communicating with each other through the 'gaps' in their cell membranes, exchanging cytoplasmic contents, primarily sodium, potassium and chloride. Why does it happen? Because these electrically charged ions move in and out of the cell altering the electrical charge of the cell's interior. As I said a while ago, this change in voltage gradient across cell membrane is a signal for ion channels to open or shut and therefore has the potential to conduct a signal. That is why the isolated cells also need the salt in the medium, which allows cells to use this salt to maintain or alter the electrical environment. It is almost like the isolated cells are running on a battery. Do you know that your batteries have such salt solutions with positive and negative charges!! It is the same principle.

Incredible, isn't it?

In fact, even the whole heart beats non-stop when separated from the body if kept in the right solution. I have seen a frog's heart placed in saline beat autonomously even when it is isolated from the frog's body! This is because the inbuilt signal generator is intact. Even the human heart can beat alone, separated from the body, if kept in the right medium. That is why heart transplant is possible.

Basically, what happens in the intact heart is the electrical impulse from the primordial signal generator, the sino-atrial node, depolarises the cell membrane. This means that the negative charge of the inside of the cells is decreased due to movement of the ions across the cell membrane, through voltage-gated ion channels we talked about a while ago.

This triggers an action potential in the heart muscle cells resulting in a contraction. Sodium, Potassium and Chloride are the three essential players in this life's most fundamental process. Sodium and Potassium are positively charged. Chloride is negatively charged. These three elements keep moving in and out of the cell in a systematic manner, assisted by a cell membrane-bound molecular pump.

Cell's interior is normally negative. The net negative charge of the cell's interior is a result of the balance between negatively charged elements and positively charged elements. In other words., cell's interior is predominated by more of negatively charged elements compared to the positively charged elements. That is why the interior of the cell is negative.

When the heart muscle cell is ready to be stimulated for contraction, there is an influx of Sodium atoms from the outside of the cell to the inside. There is some inward movement of negatively charged Chloride atoms also. Sodium and Chloride are more abundant outside the cell compared to the interior. During this process the Potassium atoms move out of the cell's interior to the outside. Potassium is more abundant inside the cell compared to the outside. The ATP-driven molecular pump which helps in shifting these atoms inside and outside act such that there is an excess of positively charged atoms moving into the cell making the cell's interion positive. When this change in the electrical potential reaches a critical level, the cell responds with a pre-programmed stimulation and the technical name for this is 'action potential'. When this point is reached there is enough power to initiate and sustain the contraction of the heart muscle cell. Once stimulated and contracted the heart muscle cell undergoes a reversal of the atom movement and the cell's interior becomes negative again. Then the next cycle begins. In a minute there are 72 such stimulations and contractions working totally automatically.

I said a while ago that isolated heart muscle cells can exhibit the same stimulation and contraction (without their rhythm generator sino-atrial node) if the isolated heart muscle cell is placed in a salt solution. Salt solutions (Saline) consists of Sodium and Chloride. This is reminiscent of the sea water, and it must be noted that life systems evolved in the sea. Despite 3500 million years the life systems cannot find a better alternative to salt for life functions. Technically speaking batteries work on the same principle.

Batteries create electricity to do physical work by moving electrons from one metal (Anode, electron-rich) to another metal (Cathode, electron-poor) connected through an electric circuit. For the reaction to work something positively charged also must move from the anode to the cathode to balance the negatively charged electrons. This comes from the electrolyte solution that must be housed inside the battery in the form of a liquid or solid.

Before we move on, it is necessary to point out here that for the same reason Sodium, Potassium, Chloride concentrations in our body is vitally important to support the battery-like function of the heart cells. If you run out of Sodium or potassium or Chloride, the 'heart cell battery' is drained. It will not work. Your heart stops beating. That is why one of the most fundamental cellular homeostatic processes involves maintenance of the right cellular concentrations of the salt solutions. There are exquisite control mechanisms that aim to restore the constancy of the electrolyte solutions. When this fails the body enters a diseased state and often the outcome is terminal cessation of life because of the vital role played by the salt elements in cellular excitation. A traveller getting caught in a desert has very little time left to live. Loss of the precious salt solutions in the sweat leads to a precariously low level of the salt solution inside the cells. The Heart muscle cell contraction stops just as your car battery ran out of the electrolyte solution.

The sequence of events is so like ordinary muscle contractions in the rest of the body (i.e., skeletal muscle). In the case of contraction of skeletal muscles like hand or legs, the stimulus comes from the brain in the form of an electrical stimulus or a neurotransmitter molecular message like acetylcholine. But the movement of electrically charged atomic elements across the cell membrane is the same as in the heart muscle cell.

In the heart this stimulus comes from intrinsically generated electrical impulses within the heart whereas the stimulus for the skeletal muscle cell comes from the brain according to a goal-oriented locomotion plan.

Defects in generation of intrinsic electrical signals in the heart can result in abnormal heart rhythms. This can happen in conditions, apart from inadequate electrolytes, where there is damage to heart muscle such as lack of blood supply (heart attack), inflammation, enlargement etc. Physical damage to the heart muscle cells can result in improper heart contraction.

II. The Central Command

Let us look at the brain now. We all know that the brain stores your information in the form of memories. We still do not have a full understanding of how this is achieved by the brain. The brain processes all your day-to-day social information and I have referred to this and its relationship to possible diseases in the decoder category as well.

The brain is said to be the control centre of our body. It can control the actions of all your body parts. Based on input from your sensory receptors situated all over the body the brain 'decides' to act. The sensory receptors communicate to the brain through the nerves. The brain can take rational decisions and send commands to respective body parts. If you have a problem the brain tells you what to do. If you are faced with a threat the brain tells you what to do. The brain tells you when to eat, when to procreate and when to sleep. The brain also tells you when to cry and when to laugh as the emotions are under its control.

The brain has several control centres typical of a cybernetic system. These control systems would depend on incoming information (input) to process the information and an output will be sent out which will be usually some sort of command to a part of the body concerned with a dedicated function. The brain has a 'Thirst centre' that controls your thirst sense indirectly controlling your body fluid balance, a 'Satiety centre' that tells you when to eat and when to stop eating which directly controls your energy balance, a 'breathing centre' that directly controls your respiration and thereby influencing availability of the vital oxygen, an 'emotion centre' situated in the limbic system part of the brain that takes you through the motions of melancholy and despair and you can go on telling more and more.

A specialised part of the brain called the respiratory centre in the brain, represented by groups of neurons situated in the medulla oblongata and pons at the base of the brain, repetitively fire due to their intrinsic nature.

This is so like the ability of the heart to generate impulses intrinsically. The same set of battery-like reactions happen here in the brain respiratory centre too. This requires movement of electrically charged (positive and negative) elements across the cell membranes of these nerve cells inside the respiratory centre of the brain. The nerve cells excite each other, and no nerve section or brainstem lesion can abolish this rhythmic excitation.

This respiratory centre is modulated by afferent (incoming) information sensed by chemoreceptor cells in carotid and aortic bodies (which sense the oxygen concentration) and carried by Vagus and Glossopharyngeal nerves, as well as information sensed by the stretch receptors in bronchi and bronchioles carried by the Vagus nerve. That is why we see variations in our breathing rate depending on the situations. When we are in danger we hyperventilate—meaning the rate of breathing increases presumably to increase the intake of oxygen. Drugs such as opiates, sodium valproate and anaesthetics can cause respiratory depression by affecting the neuronal activity in the respiratory centre leading to depression of the central nervous system (coma) due to lack of oxygen. Acute brain oedema due to concussion and brain damage can also affect the electrical activity-generating capacity of the respiratory centre.

III. DNA Blueprint

Then we move on to the more obvious DNA as the basis for derangement of cellular information. Alteration in the information content of the DNA due to damage by physical, biological and chemical agents, or due to errors in DNA replication or genetic inheritance, is an obvious cause of disease.

It could be a chromosomal defect (e.g., Down's syndrome) a monogenic defect (e.g., Cystic Fibrosis) or due to specific mutations (e.g., Sickle cell anaemia). Or gene mutations can result in diseases like Phenylketonuria, Albinism etc.

Many types of cancers are now known to be a result of mutations in important control genes.

The cells go out of control because these mutations destroy the information present in those genes. Often, it takes only a tiny change in the gene sequences to completely affect the information they encode. It is no different from corrupt files in your computer. It is like an error in the program codes that control your machines. The body 'machine' is so robustly built that it can withstand several less significant 'coding errors' without ceasing to function.

That is why many gene mutations in different organs cause diseases that are not instant killers. There is so much redundancy and resilience built in our bodies that minor to moderately severe errors can be tolerated. Usually, there are alternate solutions that will come to the rescue.

It is now suspected that even susceptibility to chronic infectious diseases could be genetically determined. In other words, people get infected because they lack the capacity to fight these infections. This ability to stand against the microbes is determined by the genes, which code for antibodies and associated 'molecular weapons' such as interferons and complement.

This immune capacity is determined at the population level in the form of herd immunity. COVID outbreaks starkly illustrated this phenomenon.

There are so many other diseases including Cancer that have been shown to be due to errors in gene codes. These errors in the gene codes lead to improper cell functions. Thanks to the human genome sequencing project, which helped to decipher the human DNA, we now know of hundreds of such gene associations with diseases. Not long ago we only thought genetic diseases like chromosomal abnormalities only led to diseases.

In short, diseases due to defects in information source would be comparable to central server problems or database corruption.

B. Coding, Transmission and Channel Errors

This category refers to problems that can arise in the generation of encrypted information.

What I mean here is the error (s) that can occur in the transmission of the information between communicating cells. As Shannon stressed in his theory, the capacity of a communication system to handle the information can be measured. He showed that a communication system has a certain 'bandwidth', signal power, and will have to deal with noise.

If the rate of information transfer is within these limits of the ability of the communication system, then information transfer can be done with little error. Though, as said earlier, Shannon applied this mathematical relationship to electrical signal transfer people have seen the relevance of the same principles to all modes of information transfer, including biology.

I can see that a defect in the nerve compromises its capacity to transmit the impulse, which is basically a channel error.

This is like problems in our modern fibre-optic telecommunication cables. A defect in a hormone production for example is a coding error in Shannon's terms. A defect in the hormone receptor is going to compromise the decoding of the biological message and if Shannon is right will impact on the ability of the body to respond to the biochemical signals. In terms of the effect of this reduced or defective information transmission it depends on the hormone system affected. As a doctor I can see it as a disease.

Even though DNA is indeed the source of all cellular information the actual cellular communication is not through the

DNA form.

Instead, the DNA information is converted into informational molecules like the hormones, growth factors and neurotransmitters etc. This is like percolation of governmental decisions from top down. The decisions taken by the ministers are first communicated to the bureaucrats who then transmit the information to the common man. It never happens the prime minister directly communicates his or her decision to you and me.

I. Information Highway

Equally important is the conduction of electrical signals from specialised cell types in your body like brain and heart to individual organs down the information cables like nerves and spinal cord.

The nerves and spinal cord are like information highways through which information travels from command centres to cellular soldiers. They are like hotlines.

Nerve palsies and disease such as Poliomyelitis are clear examples where the nerves are malfunctioning. In the case of Polio, the cause is the poliovirus, which damages the nerve ganglions in the spinal cord. In the case of nerve palsies there are several causes including viruses, metabolic conditions like diabetes, physical damage etc.

Multiple Sclerosis is one well-known nerve disease where problems in insulation of the nerve lead to inability to conduct electrical signals correctly.

II. Coded Messages to the Cellular Subjects

The other major problem arises due to errors in generation of coded messages like hormones. A 'hormone' or a 'growth factor' or a 'neurotransmitter' is like a software program generated by a command organ/tissue that is 'run' by the target cells to elicit a defined biological program. To do that the respective target cells will have to first 'sense' the release of the 'molecular code' through their cell-surface 'molecular aerials' called receptors.

Due to various types of physical, biological or chemical insults hormone-secreting organs like pituitary, thyroid gland, adrenal glands, pancreas, parathyroid gland etc. can become affected. The result is failure to produce these hormones or growth factors. As mentioned before the hormones are very important informational molecules controlling vital biological programs ranging from growth, reproduction, metabolism etc.

For example, lack of thyroid hormone can lead to hypothyroidism which basically means an underactive thyroid. Goitre refers to enlargement of the thyroid gland and can occur with hypothyroidism, hyperthyroidism, or normal thyroid function.

The opposite is also true.

Overproduction of thyroid hormones is also not good. Problems in generation of informational molecules, like in endocrine deficiency states, such as inability to make hormones like cortisol and aldosterone due to adrenal disease, inability to make growth hormone due to pituitary disease, inability make insulin leading to diabetes, inability to make thyroxine in thyroid disease, inability to produce sex hormones due to gonadal disease etc. can be huge medical problems sometimes needing life-long treatments.

III. Wrong Signal at the Wrong Time

Sometimes, such hormonal molecules can be produced at the wrong times by the wrong organs. The most common situation when this is likely to occur is cancer. Cancer cells, by virtue of their ability to de-differentiate and re-differentiate, acquire the unwanted capacity to make hormones and growth factors, which they are not supposed to produce.

Because the source of these molecules is from an abnormal location it is often referred to as ectopic production. But the problem is that wherever these molecules are produced the effects are the same. Inappropriate signalling due to generation of informational molecules by cancers (ectopic hormones, growth factors etc.), activation/deactivation of regulatory genes affecting the information flow (inactivation of tumour suppressor genes, inappropriate activation of growth factor/mitogenic factors by oncogenes etc.) can lead to a variety of disease conditions.

This is like forcing the cells to take biochemical actions not consistent with the metabolic state of the cells and tissues. Because these molecular signalling codes are impersonal. The release of the codes will bring about the expected action and there is no one to sit and analyse whether these codes are appropriate or not. Basically, the body is confused by the release of molecular signals that are not appropriate to the situation.

I guess I must use some common examples to explain the above paragraph. For the non-medical readers, it may not be readily apparent what this means. What would you do, or what would you expect your government to do, to deal with poverty? I suppose you would expect the governments to take actions that will help distribute resources to the needy.

On the contrary, if the government took actions that led to the direct opposite i.e., more accumulation of wealth in the hands of a few privileged people, this is like the inappropriate signalling in cellular parlance that leads to disease. The fact is this is not a totally hypothetical example. It is a real-life example where things are appropriately handled. Another example I can think of is the decision taken by governments to go to war at enormous expense when there are millions of people starved of food, water or other amenities like schools, hospitals. I do not think any reader will think this is an implausible example.

IV. Hacking Cellular Information

Poisoning is a common medical problem which doctors face in their routine practice. Effects of various poisons and venoms produced by snake, fish, insects etc. can lead to blockade/inappropriate activation of several human physiological processes like axonal conduction affecting neural transmissions, mast cell activation leading to anaphylactic reactions (or anaphylactoid reactions in some contexts), cardiac rhythm disturbances, neuromuscular conduction resulting in paralysis etc.

Poisons really affect our information conduction channels. Can you believe that? A snake bite for example can paralyze us. Do you know why? The snake poison hits our neuromuscular junctions and interferes with the communication of messages from the nerves to the muscles by hitting the acetylcholine receptors. Because of that your muscles cannot contract and because your muscles cannot contract you cannot run or even move.

The result is that you lie there helplessly while your attacker consumes you. Some snake venoms can cause paralysis of your heart muscle such that you will be starved of blood circulation. Some snake venoms can interfere with your blood coagulation so that you will bleed to death! They do that by disabling the molecular information flow in the coagulation cascade.

Coagulation is a multi-step process where successive molecular actions are required for the next step to start. If you block one step, then the whole sequence gets derailed. Snake poisons can do exactly that by interfering with the regulated blood clotting process.

The interference from the snake poison will make it difficult for the blood to clot. Consequently, you bleed to death. Doctors use blood clot-busting drugs to dissolve blood clots. If you use these drugs excessively, then the patient starts to bleed. Snake poisons can derail the orderly function of the double-edged sword i.e., maintaining a liquid blood. It is really shocking to note that the poisonous animals are hacking into the communication channels in our body to cause death.

They intercept our normal communications between cells to bring about disruption.

V. Hijacking the Cell

Viruses in general have an ability to interfere with our protein synthesis function. What does this mean? It means they, despite being invisible, can block the translation of DNA blueprint in our cells so that our cells are deprived of our executable codes.

The cells are simply unable to function the usual way. This is because the viruses hijack the ribosomal apparatus and the rest of the protein synthesis machinery of our cells. This means that our own cellular proteins cannot be made using the DNA transcripts.

These DNA transcripts are read by the ribosomes and according to the DNA code the individual amino acid 'alphabets' are assembled no different from how we use English alphabets to construct meaningful sentences.

Proteins are 'molecular sentences' constructed as messages using the DNA blueprint. Viruses hijack our protein synthesis machinery and make their protein products at the expense of our products. This is incredible. All types of viruses do the same including the Corona-SARS virus that is holding the world to ransom now. Even though the DNA itself is intact and even the transcription of genes is normal it is the next step in the information process that is affected.

Depending on the organ infected by the viruses a variety of diseases can result.

Viruses are information hackers to the core! There are so many viruses out there each with a unique way of hacking into our cellular protein synthesis in their target organs. There are viruses for every type of organ. There are hepatitis viruses causing liver impairment (Jaundice), viruses that affect the brain (encephalitis and meningitis), there are viruses that affect the nerves (Polio), viruses that affect the lung (causing pneumonia) and so on. In all cases the modus operandi is similar.

C. Decoding (Receiver) Errors

Defects in information capture and processing of cellular information can result due to several reasons. The primary problem is that the receiver cell is unable to make sense of the message either because it was not received correctly or because it was not processed correctly.

It is like the difference between speaking a language that you know and speaking one that you do not know. Your brain will not be able to process any of the words that you hear if you do not know the language. It is easy to see the effects of brain malfunction causing psychiatric or neurological problems. Neuronal information processing defects can be due to organic damage to parts of central nervous system or due to tumours, toxins, infections like meningitis, encephalitis etc. or lack of energy or oxygen supply or lack of sodium or potassium affecting the electrical activity of the neurons.

I wonder whether death is the effect of inability to capture vital information or is the cause of it, if you know what I mean. Give it a thought. I always find it fascinating to think about.

Coma is the state in which an individual loses the ability to respond to information from the external world but not his internal world. They can keep their blood pressure under control, have blood at a stable pH, keep breathing to keep their oxygen concentration etc. It is true that they may need help with medical assistance in the form of life support machines to do so. It is yet incredible that his or her 'cellular society' is largely intact as far as information exchange is concerned, within the internal world of his. But he or she is dead to the outside world.

This is because none of the externally generated information like sound, smell, vision etc., reach the brain of the comatose individual.

I. Cellular Offices

I said earlier that cells do a lot of decoding function. They receive a variety of cellular messages, and these messages must be properly deciphered. The receptors and their ligands work like lock and key. They snugly bind each other to throw open the entry points of information across the cell membrane.

In every sense of the word a cell-surface receptor can be compared to an office receptionist. The receptionist can greet visitors and decide if they are to be let through to meet your office staff or they should be stopped at the entrance and only their messages can be taken in by another office staff. In many cases cells transmit the incoming messages to the inside of the cell by passing on the primary message to a secondary messenger. It is equally true that there can be a third-level messenger which will be involved for the final transfer of information to the actual effector. This is almost like a relay race where the baton is passed onto successive runners.

For example, a hormone message will need a specific receptor to decipher the message. If this receptor is defective, due to a gene mutation etc. then the cell will be unable to properly read the hormone signal. This is a typical example of what is called a hormone resistance state. Though your body made the hormone signal it becomes ineffective. Its job cannot be done. If the hormone in question can be considered as insulin, for example, the person becomes a diabetic because his body cells cannot 'read' the insulin program because of the insulin receptor defect. The hormone gene is fine and so is the ability of the concerned cell to make the hormone, but the receptor molecule is the culprit. Several diseases result due to such errors. The defect is in the hormone receptor which fails to act as a decoder. The outcome is an improper signal capture when the respective hormone signal binds the receptor. Many diseases are known to result due to such hormonal decoding defects such as insulin resistance, thyroid hormone resistance, testicular feminisation syndrome due to androgen receptor defect, Nephrogenic Diabetes Insipidus due to anti-diuretic hormone

(ADH) receptor resistance etc.

In the case of insulin resistance, the hormone insulin is available in plenty, but they are ineffective. So, the cells act as if there is no insulin signal is around. The problem is the decoding inability of insulin receptor. Because insulin is not acting effectively, though available in plenty, the outcome is like insulin deficiency we see in diabetes mellitus. In the case of testicular feminisation syndrome, the male sex hormone receptor is not able to decode the signal associated with the androgen, the male sex hormone. So, the biological effect of masculinity goes missing. The patients tend to become 'feminized' due to unopposed action of the female sex hormones.

II. Crosstalk in Cell-Cell Communication can be Bad

Defects in cellular decoding can also arise if there is a 'Crosstalk' due to very similar informational molecules interacting with signal transduction machinery of each other resulting in unwanted, unintended activation of events often leading to cellular dysfunction. This is like the cross talk between two telephone lines when you can hear the conversation between two people you have no business with. An example is the autoimmune disease that arises due to antibodies directed against microbial antigens going off target. The misguided, 'cross-talking' antibodies hit the host cell antigens due to antigenic similarity. Classic example of this crosstalk is the Rheumatic heart disease, which results due to similarity between one of the molecules on the surface of the bacterium Streptococcus and a protein on the heart muscle. The antibody made by the patient, targeting the staphylococcus bacteria, veer off course and hit the patient's own heart muscle cells. Due to this 'cross-fire' heart muscle cells die. The patient develops heart disease.

III. Forged Cellular Passports

Other types of examples for crosstalk would be the origin of infectious diseases due to microbial entry into host cells through receptor uptake/internalisation pathways meant for host molecules. This again happens due to the confusion of structural similarities.

An example is again Staphylococcus aureus, which is known to cause pustular skin infections. They have receptors for binding human tissue connective tissue proteins like fibronectin, laminin, collagen, fibrinogen. Why would bacteria have these receptors that can bind human connective tissue proteins? That is a philosophical question to ask. Regardless of the philosophy the outcome of this bizarre phenomenon is that these bacteria can bind the human connective tissue proteins.

As a result, entry of these harmful bacteria into the connective tissue is allowed where they stay happily. Once inside these bacteria flourish and cause the infections. Because of the location of the infection these bacteria cause predominantly skin infections.
Another example would be the case of the bacteria that causes Leprosy, called Mycobacterium leprae, which binds host cell fibronectin potentiating entry into nerve cells and skin cells. As we know leprosy bacteria have the affinity for nerves and skin and that is why the manifestations of this disease are unsightly.

IV. Using Molecular Information to Stab Microbes to Death

Disruptive strategies of microbes which interfere with signal decoding by immune cells can lead to immune evasion by the microbes and the consequent infectious disease.

What this means is that microbes can prevent proper information exchange between our cells which are actively involved with fighting the microbes.

What would happen in such a case?

The immune cells would not know where to hit the microbe. In a typical immune attack, our body cells (lymphocytes and neutrophils) should be able to know about the nature of the enemy microbes so that they can initiate an attack that is powerful and suitable for the microbe in question.

The attack could consist of development of antibodies or other 'molecular weapons' like interferons and interleukins.

To make precise, custom-fit antibodies the immune cells should talk to each other and exchange the information about the identity of the microbe.

I suppose this is like the need for sharing information between different law enforcement organisations when they fight criminals and terrorists. Countries often share information between each other for the purpose of fighting crime.

With respect to our human body, a microbe is a criminal and we need to fight it. But the criminals—like microbes—perform counter-espionage actions to not only know of the attack against them but often they are able to corrupt the intelligence information gathered by the immune cells. Apologies for using such an anthropomorphic language but I am helpless. Microbe do spoil our immune efforts by counter-intelligence measures, whether you want to believe it not.

One type of immune attack is called the complement-mediated cell death. A cascade of reactions is initiated by a variety of proteins called complement proteins by the immune process. The outcome of this complement activation is formation of a hollow-core, tube-like molecular structure that gets inserted on the cell wall of the microbial culprit (not entirely unlike stabbing).

It is like assembling a weapon only when it is needed.

Consequently, the microbial cell wall gets leaky, and all cellular contents leak out killing the microbe. This is amazing. I think this is no different from the way we kill by shooting bullets that put holes on your body! Complement system is an effective and powerful weapon in our immune armoury!

While it is already unbelievable for the readers that our

immune cells stab the microbes to death, I guess it is likely to be equally incredible that the microbes know a trick or two how to evade the knife stabbing or the antibody bullet?

The microbes can either coat them with a layer of molecules that will shield their surface (like a bullet-proof vest or the ancient armour) or use decoys such that your bullets and the arrows follow the lifeless decoy molecule instead of the real microbe!

V. Molecular Camouflage to Escape the Wrath of Targeted Cellular Missiles:

An example of microbial interference in immune cell information transfer is the case where Lipopolysaccharide (LPS), a type of endotoxin produced by Gram-negative bacteria like Salmonella (causative agent for Typhoid), Shigella (which causes dysentery), E. coli (causes diarrhoea) and Neisseria meningitidis (causes Meningitis) forms a confluent layer on the bacterial surface preventing the complement-mediated cell lysis.

The effect is that your immune attack on these bacteria is nullified.

Neisseria gonorrhoeaee produces a shorter LPS with an extra sialic acid added by its own Tran sialidase, which can block complement activation. The effect is the same as above. The outcome is that these microbes go unchecked freely colonising human organs. I guess this can be compared to wearing a bullet proof jacket to evade the bullets as I said earlier.

These microbes lurk around our vicinity well prepared to give a slip to our attacks. So, diseases are to be seen as failure of our immune system to effectively counter the sleazy tricks coming from the microbes.

VI. Information Failure as the Basis of the End

Death, due to disease or injury, invariably involves a breakdown of the information network in the brain eventually. It is the direct or indirect cause of the death itself. Was it the information failure that caused the death? Or death caused the breakdown of information exchange? It is difficult to answer this question in many cases. It is like the Chicken or Egg controversy. Which comes first?

I feel looking at disease as a failure of information gives a totally different dimension to medical sciences. Diseases have never been classified before based on information. This is a totally new attempt that views diseases from a totally new perspective. For the very first time, there is a unification of the disease-causing principles under one umbrella. It makes sense to look at various diseases from this angle. Going by this medical analogy, I guess the end of humanity, if it ever comes, will be orchestrated by failure in our information networks. Our modern society has become so digitized that almost everything is now based on information exchange and processing. Whether it is banking or shopping or travel or work everything is based on communication between entities.

We take pride in making everything digital. By doing so we have made ourselves vulnerable. Just what would happen if there was a breakdown of information between people or devices? The impact would be localised or widespread. This is like a minor organ dysfunction happening due to a localised disturbance in a particular organ or tissue. Or it could be a more global impairment of body function or even death if the damage is at a more fundamental level.

Doomsday soothsayers often talk fondly of the end of the world. There is never a dearth of books discussing such possibilities. I do not want to join this band of pseudo-scientists, but my impression is some form of information failure will accompany the end of humanity without doubt. There will be a time when there is going to be a total shut down of all information networks in the world leading to utter chaos and shut down across the globe.

What if a massive sun storm hit the world frying all out electronic devices? What if the Internet collapses? What if there was a shortage of power needed to run our networks?

Anything can happen. It is my bet that the world will meet its end then.

This is the equivalent of death for a life system.

For this to happen the hit should affect some critically important processes such that recovery or restoration is not possible in the required timeframe.

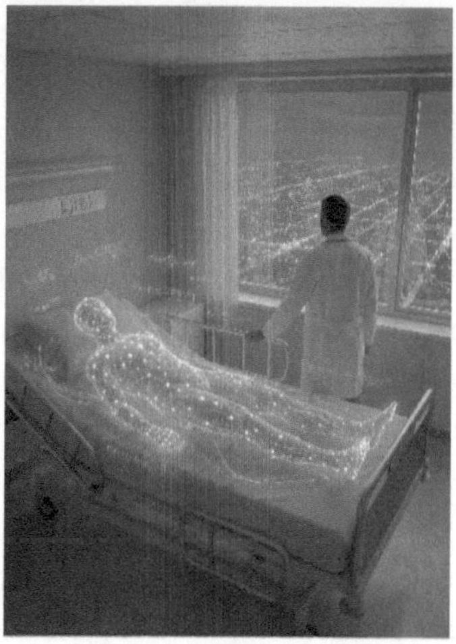

16. End Note

WE NOW COME to the end.

Are we now in a better position to understand the phenomenon of disease?

There were a few major observations I made about diseases that represent major departures from conventional teaching. These observations point to the possibility that we can find some deeper meanings for the term 'disease'. An orthodox medical professional may or may not like the way I have analysed the concept of diseases, but this attempt is to simplify the basis of human diseases for the benefit of those interested.

Firstly, I put forward the hypothesis that the human body is a society constituted by diverse cellular cultures. There are 30 trillion cells in the body which is about 4000 times more than the global human population. There are about 200 to 400 types of cells in our body, each representing a unique cellular culture.

We all know how difficult it is to live in a multicultural society. The unique thing about the human body is that all cells cooperate with each other. The culture of cellular cooperation and non-exploitation is yet to be seen in the human society. Despite the almost perfect set-up of cellular communication and cooperation inside the body there are occasional or permanent disruptions in cellular communication that lead to diseases.

The diseases are viewed as failures in the cellular society much like the social problems that we encounter. The comparison made here between social problems of our human society and diseases opens the possibility of a truly novel view of human diseases. One does not expect medical schools to teach the students likening sociological problems to diseases.

But, as I said at the outset, I wanted to explore human diseases from a fundamental point of view to identify some simple, unifying principles. This may have appeared to be an exercise that has no real value in the real world. But I said that even art has no purpose but surprisingly can give us joy and pleasure. Surprisingly, the similarities between social maladies and human diseases raises the unexpected possibility to solve social problems using medical principles.

In one whole chapter I showed how most if not all medical treatment strategies for various diseases are so much like what sociologists and politicians do to solve social issues. There are some intriguing outcomes arising out of this analogy.

Firstly, the human body operates on a communal basis where all cells in the body receive an equal share of the food delivered to their 'doorstep' through a network of blood vessels. It is said that no body cell is farther than 50 microns distance from a nearest capillary!

Where there is a need there is prioritized allocation of resources based on need rather than greed. This is unusual in our societies which is a point worth noting. Inequality in wealth is a huge social problem that is likely to test the longevity of our human societies.

Common people, as well as economists, are noticing the problems underlying the undesirable accumulation of resources by a few privileged people while most common people go starving. At the risk of appearing politically incorrect I am forced to conclude that capitalism is a disease afflicting the human society no different from the cancers. This is a startling outcome of the approach that I used to understand human diseases. It is not what I was trying to prove or something. It just emerged as an off-shoot idea that is intriguing to say the least.

In the same vein, I make the daring statement that we will never get rid of terrorism from our world how much ever national governments try. It is a manifestation of an ageing society. There is saying that 'familiarity breeds contempt'. That is what happens when cells lose their tolerance towards their own 'cellular compatriots'. Despite exquisite mechanisms within the body to condone autoimmune attacks on cells by fellow 'citizen cells' we still find 'cellular terrorism'. Presence of autoantibodies in a significant proportion of ageing people is a sign that even the evolutionarily perfected human body has not solved the problem.

If hundreds of thousands of years of evolutionary change have not solved the riddle, then how are we going to do it with our short 5000-year history of political leadership?

The second major unifier in the understanding of human diseases is the vital importance of cellular information transfer in maintaining the state of health. A healthy state of the body means perfect cooperation between all the cells and organs for which information transfer is critical.

When the information transfer between body cells does not happen properly then there is disorderly function of the body either in a localized or widespread manner. I used Shannon's information theory framework to show how the body as a communicating system fits perfectly in this model. I also showed how every type of human disease can be understood as defects in Information source, conduction errors or deciphering errors. No disease can escape this simple classification which is remarkable to say the least. No medical textbook of any kind anywhere in the world discusses human diseases from this point of view.

The third unifying principle I have identified is the 'final common pathway to death', a phenomenon wherein diverse initial insults to the body converge on progressively fewer pathways eventually culminating in one single ride to the end. It does not matter what the initial insult was. An insult is any causative factor that causes a disturbance to the orderly function of a group of cells. It could be a microbial infection, chemical toxin, a genetic defect, a nutrient deficiency, an immunological disorder or any form of disease-causing etiological factor.

After the initial insult then the progression of the damage takes predictable routes where the nature of the initial insult does not matter anymore. After the initial convergence there is further funnelling of these fewer pathways into one single final pathway that can be viewed as the 'last journey' that moves hurriedly towards its destination point named Death.

I have shown how diverse biochemical derangements affecting essential elements lead to more pervasive damage to vital processes which, in turn, have collective effects on one or two indispensable, life-sustaining properties. Invariably, the final common pathway impacts on oxygen supply and all people who die will do so because their body cells failed to procure, deliver and supply oxygen for production of energy for running the body machine. Lack of oxygen delivers the literal death blow! Before undertaking this irreversible, one-way journey the body goes about the long and protracted route of multiple disease processes caused by innumerable etiological agents.

Obviously, we do not die every day. Death is once in a lifetime event! Under normal circumstances it happens after 70 or 80 years which means that we have managed to avoid undertaking this one-way, final journey for so long!

That means we have many safety mechanisms to bail us out of difficult situations that can potentially make us embark on our last trip each time. But we survive. When the internal homeostatic mechanisms fail our doctors come to our rescue. Much of our treatment strategies, I showed, are aimed at restoring homeostatic balance. Continuing with the theme of homeostatic balance I alluded to the comparison of the human body to a cybernetic system in one of the earlier chapters. Viewing the human diseases as failures in one or more of the sensors in the cybernetic system which results in inability to adapt to fluctuations in the internal environment is a unifying concept that throws a different light on the nature of the human diseases.

The human body is a thermodynamic system talking in strictly physical terms. It is an open system. An open thermodynamic system is defined as a system that takes in something and leaves out something. There is an inward flow of matter as well as an outward one. The outward flow can include, apart from other things, simple heat. We fulfil the definition of an open thermodynamic system to the letter. We eat food which is what continuously feeds matter into the body while it functions as a thermodynamic system. Food is combusted in presence of oxygen to produce free energy as well as wasteful heat. Food is also the source of essential elements for conducting metabolism and growth. We excrete waste products back into the environment and we also emit heat that is wasted. Emission of wasteful heat is one of the hallmarks of a thermodynamic system.

When we die our body becomes a closed thermodynamic system. It is unable to take in matter nor can it put out matter/heat. Whatever that existed inside the human body, in terms of chemical elements and molecules, come under the strict control of laws governing chemistry and physics.

Biology is destroyed and chemistry and physics take over the control of the lifeless body. The matter that was associated with your human body is now just a physicochemical asset held by the planet. It is no more yours. The order that was associated with the biological organization of the human body is disassembled with the assistance of the microbial scavengers to return the chemical elements back to useable form for the benefit of the Mother Nature. The microbes transiently metabolize the matter inside your dead body as used goods before there are returned to the environment. This matter will be recycled too.

The point to be noted is that in the dead state we are unable to carry out directed, useful, metabolic reactions due to lack of energy. Instead, the chemical elements simply follow the Law of Mass action wherein a set of reactants enter a chemical reaction to form the products.

The build-up of the products will reverse the reaction in the opposite way till the concentration of the reactants reach a critically high concentration when the reaction will start proceeding in the forward reaction and this cycle goes on endlessly. Chemists call this a reversible reaction and biologists would call it a futile cycle.

The dead body is full of such futile, reversible reactions that do not contribute to the order that was seen in the living state. Instead, there is progressive movement of the system towards the state of disorder which is mandated by the Second Law of Thermodynamics. The Second Law of Thermodynamics states that a system would prefer to reach the state of equilibrium which is the state where maximum amount of the futile, reversible reactions happen. In other words, the equilibrium state represents the state of maximum disorder.

Life systems can contravene the Second Law of Thermodynamics and create order at the expense of food energy. That is why we eat. Eating provides us the necessary fuels and nutrients to keep the reactions move forward and not reverse. Otherwise, matter would have relentlessly moved towards the state of disorder as dictated by the Second Law.

I consider disease as a progressive inability of the human body to defy the Second Law of Thermodynamics. Endpoint is death when living matter associated with your body equilibrates with non-living matter outside.

This is my definition of disease! This is a novel view of diseases and that no medical school teaches their students this.

Finally, I propose that a disease is a multi-cellular characteristic not limited to human life systems. Various animals have been shown to seek medicinal remedies in the forests to alleviate their diseases. That raises a philosophical question—is fighting disease a survival tool? We should not forget the point that ancient humans had practiced various forms of healing to cure their diseases. This was way before the advent of science and medicine. We were no different from animals then. Wisdom had brought us several medicinal remedies that surprisingly have a scientific basis. Occurrence of innumerable medicinal agents out there in nature makes us wonder if they exist with a purpose—to heal us.

It is almost as if Nature anticipated the origin of diseases and sought to provide a solution to it.

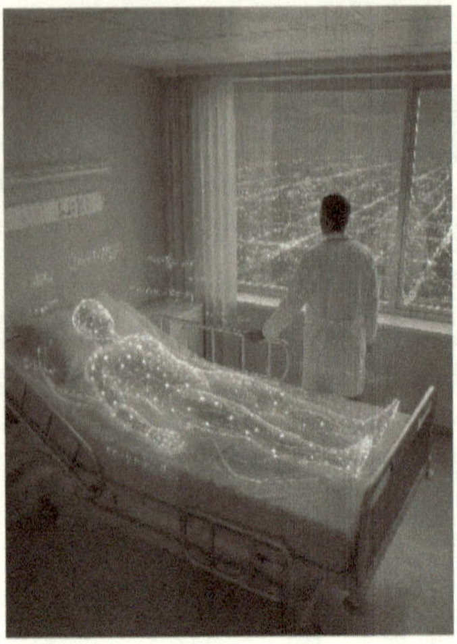

17. Appendix: Shannon Information Theory Model as Applied to the Understanding of Human Disease

THIS APPENDIX IS deliberately added for readers with a medical background without holding back any medical terminology. I thought this is the only way I can make a focussed attempt to list all types of diseases as I want in order to classify them. Those readers, particularly doctors, who have prior knowledge of human diseases, will surely benefit from this appendix. I have shied away from the conventional classification of diseases and used my own scheme. Non-medical readers may find this tough going but for your benefit I have devoted a separate chapter in the main body of the book where I have tried to explain the concept in a toned-down way.

Based on the concept of Shannon's model, it can be deduced that errors in information transmission within the human body can occur due to:

A. Defects in Information Source

Defects in generation of intrinsic electrical signals (as in cardiac arrhythmias) or faults in rhythmic signal generation as pulsatile release of hormones like ACTH, gonadotrophins (menstrual disorders) etc. and/or circadian rhythm disturbances would represent cellular dysfunction due to changes at the level of the source of information. Alteration in the information content of the DNA due to damage by physical, biological and chemical agents or due to errors in DNA replication or genetic inheritance is an obvious cause of disease.

B. Coding, Transmission and Channel Errors

Errors in transmitting the information which in the biological context would mean a) errors in neuron-to-neuron transmissions, b) errors in neuro-muscular transmissions, c) inappropriate signalling due to generation of informational molecules by cancers (ectopic hormones, growth factors etc.), activation/deactivation of regulatory genes affecting the information flow (inactivation of tumour suppressor genes, inappropriate activation of growth factor/mitogenic factors by oncogenes etc. d) effects of various poisons (produced by snake, fish, insects etc.) that lead to blockade/inappropriate activation of a number of human physiological processes like axonal conduction affecting neural transmissions, mast cell activation leading to anaphylactic reactions (or anaphylactoid reactions in some contexts), cardiac rhythm disturbances, neuromuscular conduction resulting in paralysis etc. e) problems in generation of informational molecules like in endocrine deficiency states (inability to make hormones like cortisol and aldosterone due to adrenal disease, inability to make growth hormone due to pituitary disease, inability to make thyroxine in thyroid disease, inability to make sex hormones due to gonadal disease etc.), f) errors in encoding the information through gene transcription into messenger RNA g) translation of messenger RNA into protein sequences, h) post-translational modifications such as glycosylation, methylation, acetylation that generally add informational value to the molecules such as site-directed export of newly synthesised molecules (e.g. Mannose-6-phosphate tag on lysosome-targeted enzymes the deficiency of which results in I-cell disease), and helps in recognition of receptors and enzymes etc. Oligosaccharide chains of glycoproteins play a role in signal recognition in molecular interactions also therefore qualify as mechanisms of conducting the information and i) lack of cofactors such as vitamins, minerals that are needed for enzymes that block the intermediary metabolic pathways and therefore interfere with flow of metabolic information.

C. Decoding (Receiver) Errors

Defects in information capture and processing of information can result due to a) 'Cross-talk' due to very similar informational molecules interacting with signal transduction machinery of each other resulting in unwanted, unintended activation of events often leading to cellular dysfunction (e.g. autoimmune disease due to antibodies directed against microbial antigens targeting host cell antigens due to antigenic similarity, and infectious diseases due to microbial entry into host cells through receptor uptake/internalisation pathways meant for host molecules because of structural similarities b) disruptive strategies of microbes which interfere with signal de-coding by immune cells resulting in immune evasion c) defects in hormone receptors and/or associated signal transduction systems leading to improper signal capture when the respective hormone binds (e.g. insulin resistance, thyroid hormone resistance, testicular feminisation syndrome due to androgen receptor defect, nephrogenic diabetes insipidus due to antidiuretic hormone (ADH) receptor resistance etc.), d) neuronal information processing defects due to organic damage to parts of central nervous system or due to toxins or lack of energy or oxygen supply or lack of sodium or potassium affecting the electrical activity of the neurons.

Classification of Human Disease-Causing Processes According to the Model of a Typical Shannon Information System

---

In the few paragraphs below, I have tried to classify all types of human diseases into three broad headings:

I. Diseases due to defects in information source.
II. Diseases due to coding, transmission errors.
III. Diseases due to decoding errors.

It is as simple as that.

What I am saying is that all types of diverse diseases afflicting man are explainable within one single framework of information transmission and its problems.

This type of reasoning and analysis has never been done before. What looks like an endless rant in the next few pages actually look simple when you view them in light of the above three classes of diseases which again can be confined into one single theme i.e. information failure.

Readers must pardon me and bear with the next few pages of hard medical terminology.

I have done little to even try and reduce the tone of the language so that expert readers will grasp my point.

I. Diseases Due to Alterations at the Information Source

Errors in Rhythmic Signal Generation by Excitatory Cells

Heart

Specialised cardiac cells have the capacity for self-excitation because of their lesser intracellular negativity due to their leakiness to sodium (-55 mV compared to –90 mV for most other cell types in the heart and the rest of the body). The electrical signal intrinsically originates in the sino-atrial node and travels down the inter-nodal pathways to the atrio-ventricular node, which then proceeds down the purkinje fibres to excite the ventricular muscle cells to bring about the ventricular contraction. Errors can occur in transmission, such as slow or accelerated conduction of impulses or abnormal impulse generation by non-pacemaker cells, particularly when impulse generation in sino-atrial node is absent or delayed. Ischaemic injury to cardiac tissues can cause depolarisation of cells in affected regions leading to variations in conduction velocities and areas of conduction block resulting in what is referred to as cardiac arrhythmias. Atrial and ventricular muscle diseases due to cardiomyopathy, myocarditis, rheumatic heart disease, hypertrophy of heart due to hypertensive heart disease can also lead to cardiac arrhythmias due to non-pacemaker cells taking on the role of signal generation (another example of diverse aetiologies producing common clinical outcomes). Even electrical shock to the body can upset the intrinsic electrical activity of the heart.

Respiratory Centre in the Brain

Acute brain oedema due to concussion and brain damage can affect the electrical activity of the respiratory centre in the brain, represented by groups of neurons situated in the medulla oblongata and pons at the base of the brain. These neuronal groups repetitively excite each other, and no nerve section or brainstem lesion can abolish this rhythmic excitation. This respiratory centre is modulated by afferent information sensed by chemoreceptor cells in carotid and aortic bodies (oxygen concentration) and carried by Vagus and glossopharyngeal nerves, as well as information sensed by the stretch receptors in bronchi and bronchioles carried by the Vagus nerve. Drugs such as opiates, sodium valproate and anaesthetics can cause respiratory depression by affecting the neuronal activity in the respiratory centre leading to depression of the central nervous system (coma) due to lack of oxygen.

Errors in DNA and Failure of Information Flow

Due to Chromosomal Disorders

Sex chromosomes: Turner's (45X) and Klinefelter's syndromes (47 XXY)
Autosomal chromosomes: Edward's (Trisomy 18), Down's (Trisomy 21) and Patau's (Trisomy 13) syndromes

Due to Monogenic Defects

Storage diseases: Glycogen storage diseases, Sphingolipidoses (Niemann-Pick, Gauchers, Krabbe's and metachromatic leukodystrophy), Gangliosidoses (Tay-Sachs), Mucopolysaccharidoses (Hunter's, Hurler's, Maroteaux-Lamy, Morquio)

Connective tissue disorders: diseases due to collagen biosynthetic defects (Ehlers-Danlos syndrome, Osteogenesis imperfecta, Marfan's syndrome, Cutis laxa, Pseudoxanthoma elasticum)

Cellular transport disorders: X-linked, Hypophosphataemic rickets, Hartnup disease, Cystinuria, Nephrogenic diabetes insipidus, Familial hypercholesterolemia, and Intestinal disaccharidase deficiency.

Aminoacidopathies: Phenylketonuria, Homocystinuria, Cystinosis, Alkaptonuria, Alpha-1-antitrypsin deficiency, Cystic fibrosis, Neurofibromatosis.

Due to Specific Gene Mutations

Haemoglobinopathies: Alpha-thalassemia, Sickle cell anaemia, various variant haemoglobins (e.g Hb Cranston). Disorders due to triple nucleotide repeat mutations13,14(expansion of CAG sequence within a gene leading to a sequence of polyglutamine within the coded protein): seen in Huntington's chorea, Spinocerebellar ataxia, Friedreich's ataxia, Myotonic dystrophy, Spinobulbar muscular atrophy, Fragile X mental retardation, Machado-Joseph disease, Dentatorubral-pallidoluysian atrophy).

Other Disorders Due to Specific Gene Mutations Include:

Increased risk of diseases due to specific gene mutations a) osteoporosis due to mutations in the regulatory site of type 1 collagen gene, b) Fragile X syndrome due to mutations in the flanking region of FMR1 gene, c) type 1 diabetes mellitus due to mutations in the flanking region of insulin gene, d) type 2 diabetes mellitus due to mutations in the intronic-regulatory site of Calpain 10 gene, e) breast and ovarian cancer due to mutations in BRCA 1& 2 genes, f) hereditary non-polyposis colorectal cancer due to mutations in DNA mismatch repair genes (MLH1, MSH2, MSH6, and PMS2), g) Maturity onset diabetes in the young due to mutations in MODY 1,2, and 3 genes, h) Parkinsons disease due to mutations in alpha-synuclein gene, i) thrombosis risk due to Factor V Leiden mutation, j) Colorectal cancer due to APC gene mutations, k) early-onset Alzheimer's disease due to mutations in presenilin 1,2 gene or beta-amyloid precursor protein gene, and l) late-onset Alzheimer's disease due to apolipoprotein E4 allelle, m) inactivation of tumour suppressor genes by methylation of Cytidine residues in promoter sequences resulting in human cancers, n) loss of G1 checkpoint control in cell cycle due to p53 gene mutation seen in nearly half of all human cancers, o) ras oncogene mutation seen in nearly 25% of all human cancers reducing dependence on external mitogenic signals, p) increased genetic instability (increased mutability) in human cancers due to faulty detection, repair of DNA damage due to inactivation of proteins such as p53 and faulty mechanisms to eliminate DNA damaged cells, q) Xeroderma pigmentosum due to an autosomal recessive defect in DNA repair in response to UV damage (endonuclease) increasing the susceptibility to cancer, and r) origin of cancers due to DNA damage due to chemical carcinogens (like polycyclic hydrocarbons, aromatic amines, azo dyes, nitrosamines, alkylating agents etc), radiation damage, oncogenic viruses (DNA viruses like papova, Adenovirus, Herpes, Hepadna viruses and RNA viruses like Retroviruses).

Defects in Nucleotide Biosynthesis due to Nutritional Deficiencies

Folate and vitamin B12 deficiencies can affect nucleotide

biosynthesis (critical cofactors in the nucleotide biosynthetic enzymes) and therefore affect cell multiplication due to reduced supply of raw materials for DNA synthesis and replication.

II. Diseases Due to Coding, Transmission and Channel Errors

Diseases due to Neural, Neuromuscular Channel Defects Neural Transmission Disorders:

Nerve palsies, neuritis, disorders of myelination like multiple sclerosis affecting transmission of neural impulse, degenerative damage to spinal cord, poliomyelitis etc.

Neuromuscular Disorders

a) Poisoning with Strychnine (producing muscular spasms), nerve agents such as organophosphate poisoning (muscle fasciculations due to inhibition of acetylcholinesterase activity causing an prolonged increase in acetyl choline action at the neuromuscular junction),
b) Botulism (neurotoxin released by Clostridium botulinum blocks release of acetyl choline by proteolytically cleaving synaptobrevin on the synaptic junction causing muscle paralysis),
c) Clostridium tetani, causative agent of tetanus, produces a toxin called tetanospasmin which acts at the synaptic level blocking release of inhibitory neurotransmitter resulting in continuous effects of excitatory neurotransmitter,
d) Myasthenia Gravis (auto-antibody to acetyl choline receptor blocks muscle contraction).

Diseases due to Inappropriate Signalling

a) **Stimulation/blockade of hormone action by auto-antibodies** a) Grave's disease due to thyroid stimulating hormone (TSH) receptor stimulatory antibodies mimicking the action of TSH normally secreted by pituitary gland, b) Hashimoto's disease due to thyroglobulin antibodies which cause problems in its utilization to make thyroid hormones and therefore resulting in thyroid under activity, c) Pernicious anaemia (auto-antibody to Intrinsic factor blocks its action in assisting vitamin B12 absorption).

b) **Diseases due to excessive release of informational molecules like hormones** a) Acromegaly due to secretion of inappropriately high amounts of growth hormone by pituitary, b) Cushing's syndrome due to excessive secretion of adrenocorticotrophic hormone (ACTH) by pituitary, c) Primary hyperparathyroidism due to secretion of excessive parathormone by the parathyroid glands, d) phaeochromocytoma due to overproduction of catecholamines by adrenal medulla, e) multiple endocrine neoplasia Type 1 & 2 and f) other hormonal over-activity.

c) **Diseases due to reduced secretion of informational molecules like hormones** a) Panhypopituitarism due to reduced production of pituitary hormones, b) hypothyroidism due to thyroid destruction or biosynthetic defects, c) diabetes insipidus due to inadequate secretion of anti-diuretic hormone by hypothalamus, d) defective cortisol and aldosterone production by adrenal gland due to enzymatic defects as in congenital adrenal hyperplasia, e) diabetes mellitus (Type 1) due to insulin deficiency.

d) **Diseases due to ectopic production of informational molecules by tumours inconsistent with the needs of the body** a) Hypercalcaemia of malignancy due to production of parathormone-related peptide by tumours, b) Syndrome of inappropriate ADH due to production of ADH by small cell lung cancer, lymphoma, pancreatic cancer etc. & c) Cushing's syndrome due to ectopic production of adrenocorticotrophic hormone (ACTH) by tumours.

e) **Inappropriate activation of second messengers** a) Cholera (Cholera toxin increases cyclic AMP and constitutively stimulates adenylate cyclase by ADP-ribosylating Gs protein of the adenylate cyclase complex resulting in defective fluid reabsorption in gut, b) human bladder cancer due to a single base change in v-ras oncogene coding for p21 protein which is related to a G protein with reduced GTPase activity resulting in chronic stimulation of adenylate cyclase and overproduction of cyclic AMP affecting a variety of cyclic AMP-dependent protein kinases, c) ras oncogene of murine sarcoma virus is a GTP-binding protein with GTPase activity affecting activity of adenylate cyclase, and d) gas gangrene, caused by Clostridium perfringens, is due to a toxin that has lecithinase activity which can hydrolyse phosphorylcholine on cell membrane resulting in lysis of cells.

f) **Inappropriate secretion of growth factors** Angiogenic factors (vascular endothelial growth factor and basic fibroblast growth factor) secreted by diverse tumours which attract and stimulate endothelial cells to form new blood vessels, and other mechanisms like down regulation of anti-angiogenic proteins such as thrombospondin 1 resulting in blood vessel overgrowth. Other growth-inducing agents include fms oncogene of feline sarcoma virus, which is a macrophage colony stimulating factor, sis oncogene of simian sarcoma virus which is a truncated B-chain of Platelet-derived growth factor and erb-B gene of avian erythroblastosis virus which is a truncated form of the receptor for epidermal growth factor.

g) **Altered tyrosine kinase-mediated cell signalling** Approximately half of the 20 known oncogenes of retroviruses are protein kinases, mostly of the tyrosine kinase type which can affect glycolytic enzymes, phophatidylinositol pathway in transmembrane signalling, intracellular adhesion molecule called vinculin which will determine the metastatic properties of the cancers and amplification of receptor-associated tyrosine kinase HER2/neu is seen in a considerable proportion of breast cancers and a disturbance in signalling pathways is seen in the majority of human cancers.

h) **Disordered mitogenic control by inappropriate cell signalling** Constitutive mitogenic activity due to oncogenes (ras oncogene encodes a mutant protein that releases a continuous stream of mitogenic signals into the cell), and simian virus 40 produces a viral oncoprotein such as large T antigen which allows pre-senescent cells to circumvent senescence by sequestering and inactivating pRB and p53 tumour suppressor genes.

i) **Tumorigenesis by inactivation of tumour suppressor genes** Inactivation of tumour suppressor genes, frequently by methylation of cytidine residues, leads to loss of certain mechanisms of growth control (e.g. RB1, a tumor suppressor gene associated with retinoblastoma determines entry of cells into G1 cell cycle stage).

j) **Diseases due to abnormal activation of genes due to chromosomal translocations** Burkitt's lymphoma, a tumour of B lymphocytes, results when there is a chromosomal translocation involving chromosomes 8 & 14 bringing the myc oncogene on chromosome 8 under the control of enhancer sequences for immunoglobulin genes, and chronic granulocytic leukaemia results when chromosomal translocation occurs between 9 & 22 chromosomes (Philadelphia chromosome).

Interference in Transcription/Translation of Genetic Information

a) **Poisons:** Alpha-sarcin, a fungal toxin (from Aspergillus giganteus), cleaves large RNA subunit and Ricins from castor beans are N-glycosidases that can inactivate ribosomes by cleaving a single adenine from the large subunit RNA affecting translation.

b) **Microbial toxins:** a) Diphtheria toxin inactivates elongation factor-2 by ADP-ribosylating it, preventing protein synthesis in several tissues such as throat, heart, and nerve and b) Dysentery, caused by Shigella dysenteriae, is due to the shiga toxin STX which is a N-glycosidase that can depurinate 28S and 60S ribosomal subunits halting protein synthesis44.

Defects in Flow of Information in Metabolic Pathways

a) Inborn errors of metabolism due to enzyme defects (due to mutations) represent a block in flow of information down metabolic pathways Examples include: a) Phenylketonuria due to deficiency of the enzyme phenylalanine hydroxylase, b) congenital adrenal hyperplasia due to 21 or 17-hydroxylase enzyme deficiency, c) glycogen storage diseases due to glucose 6-phosphatase or glycogen debranching enzyme deficiency, d) galactosemia due to galactokinase or galactose-1-phosphate uridyl transferase deficiency etc. These diseases are the outcomes of a failure of cell type(s) to carry out tasks such as synthesis of molecules or generation of energy in response to signals coming from other cells thereby breaking the information chain that is key to homeostatic control.

b) Metabolic diseases due to enzyme defects as a result of nutritional lack of essential co-factors like vitamins and minerals e.g. a) Pyridoxine (a cofactor for transaminases) and folic acid (vital in transfer of one-carbon moieties like methyl and methylene groups in cellular metabolism) deficiencies interfering with homocysteine metabolism causing homocystinuria, b) vitamin B12 deficiency causing methylmalonic aciduria because it is a co-factor for the methylmalonic CoA mutase enzyme, c) vitamin K deficiency affecting the coagulation cascade because it is vital for a carboxylase enzyme that carboxylates glutamate residues on prothrombin molecule which is necessary for its ability to chelate calcium, and d) vitamin A is important in post-translational glycosylation of proteins which have functional and structural roles in maintenance of mucosal cell integrity the absence of which causes night blindness, xerophthalmia and squamous dysplasia of epithelial cell lining in respiratory and urogenital tracts. The roles of minerals like calcium, phosphate, magnesium have already been discussed. Other elements like iodine (important in thyroid hormone structure) and iron (indispensable co-factor in heme moiety of the heme-containing enzymes like haemoglobin, myoglobin, catalase, tryptophan pyrrolase etc.) also need to be mentioned.

III. Decoding (Receiver Errors)

Crosstalk in Signal Transduction Machinery Leading to Autoimmune Diseases

a) antigenic cross reactivity between M protein of group A streptococci and antigens in specific human tissues such as muscle (myosin), and kidney resulting in rheumatic heart disease, and acute post-streptococcal glomerulonephritis respectively,

b) spondyloarthropathies due to anti-Klebsiella pneumoniae and anti-Shigella flexneri antibodies binding to HLA-B27 on the surface of synovial lining cells because these organisms share an arthritogenic epitope with HLA-B27 and c) other autoimmune diseases like atrophic gastritis (parietal cell antibodies), juvenile diabetes (islet cell autoantibodies), chronic active hepatitis (autoantibodies to liver-specific proteins), ulcerative colitis (autoantibodies to colon antigens), idiopathic thrombocytopenic purpura (platelet antigens), autoimmune haemolytic anaemia (red cell autoantibodies), and Goodpasture's syndrome (basement membrane autoantibodies) where the initiating culprit is less well understood.

Infectious Diseases due to Microbial Entry into Host Cells through Receptor Uptake/Internalisation Pathways meant for Host Molecules because of Structural Similarities:

Various organisms have virulence factors/attachment factors that potentiate host cell entry due to sharing of structural similarities which enable use of host cell signal recognition machinery to gain entry, e.g.

a) *Staphylococcus aureus*, which is known to cause pyogenic skin infections, have receptors for binding host tissue fibronectin, laminin, collagen, fibrinogen,
b) *Mycobacterium leprae*, the causative agent for leprosy, binds host cell fibronectin potentiating entry into Schwann cells and epithelial cells,
c) *Bordetella pertussis* binds fibronectin through its surface protein called the filamentous agglutinin,
d) *Borrelia burgdorferi*, which causes lyme disease, binds integrin $\alpha IIb\beta 3$ on human platelets,
e) *Leishmania mexicana*, causative agent of *leishmaniasis*, binds complement receptor CR3, a member of $\beta 2$ integrin family in macrophages,
f) *Adenovirus* 2 encodes 2 proteins, the fiber protein and the penton base protein, which attach to integrin receptors promoting internalisation,
g) *Entamoeba histolytica*, which causes amoebiasis, has a galactose or N-acetyl-D-galactosamine-inhibitable lectin mediating attachment of trophozoites to colonic mucins,
h) *Mycobacteria, Leishmania, Candida, Pneumocystitis Carinn*i and specific strains of enterobacteriae contain mannose-rich components within the cell wall that bind to mannose

receptors on macrophages, and

i) *Chlamydia* bind to glycosaminoglycans on host cell surface to gain entry.

Evasion of Host Immune Mechanisms by Microbes by Interfering with the Host Immune Recognition and Effector Mechanisms

a) *Lipopolysaccharide* (LPS), a type of endotoxin produced by Gram-negative bacteria like Salmonella, Shigella, E. Coli and Neisseria meningitidis forms a confluent layer on the bacterial surface preventing the complement-mediated cell lysis,
b) *Neisseria gonorrhoeae* produces a shorter LPS with an extra sialic acid added by its own transialidase which can block complement activation,
c) Strains of *Streptococci* group A bears a protein called M protein which binds the complement cascade control protein H of the host preventing its activation,
d) Proteins A & G of *Streptococci* and S. aureus both bind IgG directly preventing IgG-mediated phagocytosis,
e) *Trypomastigotes of Trypanosoma cruzi,* which causes Chagas disease (American trypanosomiasis), produces a factor which accelerates the decay of complement C3 convertases limiting complement activation,
f) *Schistosomula of Schistosoma mansoni*, the causative agent of Schistosomiasis, shed the complement-activating surface glycocalyx coat during transformation from the cercarial stage and also acquire the complement regulatory molecule called the decay-accelerating factor from the vertebral host,
g) *E. histolytica* has a multi-functional galactose-specific lectin that blocks complement-mediated killing of the organism

because of its homology with the mammalian complement inhibitor CD59,

h) *Hemophilus influenzae*, causative agent for pneumonia, secretes IgA protease-like protein,

i) *S. pneumoniae*, Candida albicans, E. histolytica produce proteases that can degrade complement C3,

j) group A *Streptococci* secrete a protease that cleaves complement chemotactic factor C5a,

k) Sialic acid-galactose-glucosamine terminal trisaccharide of the group B *Streptococcal polysaccharides* is structurally similar to a number of oligosaccharides found on mammalian glycoproteins which make them non-immunogenic, and

l) *Plasmodium falciparum trophozoites* bind thrombospondin and also members of Immunoglobulin superfamily (Intercellular adhesion molecule-1, Vascular cell adhesion molecule) and the Selectin family and to the differentiation antigen CD36 mediating attachment of the infected cell to vascular endothelium sequestering them from splenic clearance.

Hormone Resistance Syndromes due to Receptor Defects

---

a) Isolated Growth hormone deficiency due to Growth hormone mutation,

b) nephrogenic diabetes insipidus due to antidiuretic hormone resistance at the renal tubular level,

c) thyroid hormone resistance due to receptor defects,

d) testicular feminization syndrome due to androgen receptor defect,

e) leprechaunism due to insulin receptor defect,

f) familial hypercholesterolemia due to low density lipoprotein receptor defect,

g) type III hyperlipidemia due to defect in intermediate

density lipoprotein particle clearance,

h) Laron-type dwarfism due to absence of mutation of the growth hormone receptor and

i) Reaven's syndrome or Syndrome X (metabolic syndrome) due to insulin resistance.

Neurological Diseases due to Disruption in Neuronal Information Processing

---

a) Organic psychoses due to a) intra-cerebral pathology due to tumours, abscesses, haemorrhage, encephalitis, meningitis and infarction which has resulted in neuronal cell death,

b) due to metabolic disturbances like hypoxia, hyponatremia, hypernatremia, renal failure, hepatic encephalopathy, hypothyroidism (Myxoedema coma), mucopolysaccharidoses (Hunter's, Hurler's, Tay-sachs, Sandhoff's diseases) and mucolipidoses (Mannosidosis, Fucosidosis, Sialidosis), vitamin deficiency (thiamine deficiency causing Wernicke-Korsakoff psychosis), hypoglycemia,

c) drug intoxication with hypnotics, anti-depressants, LSD, amphetamines, anti-convulsants, and fungicides like organic mercurials,

d) poisoning with hallucinogenic agents like psilocybes mushrooms containing psilocin and psilocybin, cannabis and amanita muscaria poisoning (containing active principles ibotinic acid and muscimol), poisoning with volatile gases and liquids, and ethanol excess, and

e) systemic infections like malaria, HIV and pneumonia. The common principles of neuronal cell dysfunction are lack of energy (due to inadequate oxygen, fuel levels) and/or alterations in electrolytes like sodium and potassium, which affect the electrical properties of the neurons. Drugs and poisons can interfere with neuronal interactions as well by altering the balance of excitatory and inhibitory neurotransmitters and metabolic diseases like mucolipidoses cause defects in neuronal information transfer because the mucolipids like sphingomyelin, and gangliosides are crucial in binding neurons together as well as insulating the neuronal axons and dendrites preventing straying of electrical signals.

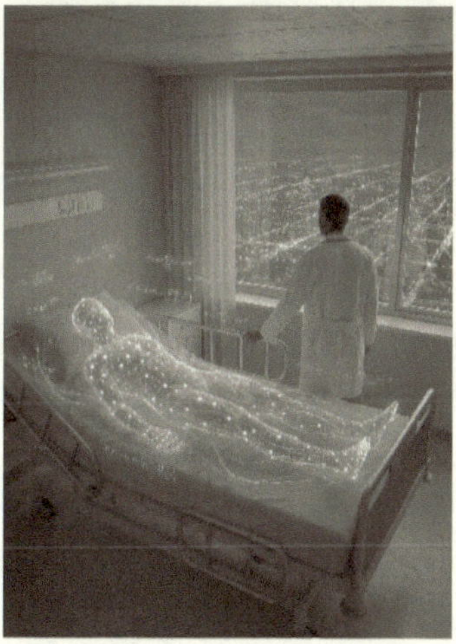

Closing Remarks

IF ANYONE CAN point out any disease that does not fit into the above framework, I will be surely surprised.

In fact, I am inclined to challenge anyone to show me a disease that does not fit in this model. I am confident that it is possible to explain all known human diseases as a defect in information exchange between cells. This can happen in various forms as shown above but the common theme of information failure is inescapable.

As I explained before, the consequence of information failure is inability to maintain the supply chain logistics inside the body. Cells suffer from the same effects that we would face in our society if we ran out of energy, food or water. Our society has a lot of restorative mechanisms to deal with resource shortages, but you will be shocked to know that it does not take much to bring the whole system down. Our body is also resilient in that sense bouncing back from disruptions but there is always a finite limit to what can be achieved when the deviations are beyond a point.

Homeostatic mechanisms are not too elastic unfortunately. They simply snap when you stretch too much. That is the point when disease and death set in.

www.ingramcontent.com/pod-product-compliance
Lightning Source LLC
LaVergne TN
LVHW100304210926
848480LV00003B/1021